To Bob, of course

Taking Care; Giving Care

Essentials for New Caregivers

Ms Joan M S Perry LICSW

ACKNOWLEDGEMENTS

I could not have written this book without the knowledge and insights I received from caregivers throughout my entire life. Although my parents and especially my mother were my primary role models, clients and friends have allowed me to see their struggles and triumphs. Some people I saw for individual counseling; others participated in caregiver support groups I facilitated; still others were and are friends and family, too numerous to mention individually. Because my work with clients is confidential, I have changed all names and identifying information and chosen to make composites of common situations and details. Thus, except for my own account, the stories I share are made from my experience in working with caregivers and care receivers and are not actual people.

Nevertheless, those caregivers and care recipients who are friends, family and clients have touched my heart, humbled me and made me a better person. I shall always be grateful for their insights and lessons. This book is a tribute not only to them and their experience, courage, and openness but to all caregivers who routinely face the same issues.

I must also acknowledge the profound influence of the two writing groups in Bradford, NH who have read page after page of my writing, helping me to eliminate detritus and paint a clearer picture and who have become a support group for me. To Sasha Wolfe, Holly Metsch, Gayle Hedrington, Lynne Lawrence and Perley Strout, and earlier to Darlene Olivo, Deborah Bernacchia and Lyn Betz, I am deeply indebted.

Thanks to Alice Kieft and Beatrice Howe who read the manuscript and provided feedback. Much gratitude to Alice who helped with the cover and thanks to Gene Seidman who designed the front of the cover.

Of course, no thanks would be complete without mentioning the Light of My Life, my husband, Bob Stauffer, whose battle with cancer and its lasting effects was lost on June 13, 2008. I am glad he was my partner and could share his sense of humor, his love and gentleness, and his beautiful soul. I am truly blessed.

Table of Contents

INTRODUCTION

On November 28th, 2000, about 10:30 in the morning, the bottom fell out of my world. Bob, my husband and anchor, the light of my life, was diagnosed with a brain tumor. I was devastated, petrified and overwhelmed. For days I went around with the deer-in-the-headlights look. I vacillated between numb and grief stricken. I functioned on autopilot. I came to believe that numb was a good state, a protective state, that enabled me to cope until I could deal with what was happening in my life. But then the waves of grief would come crashing in, unbearable and demoralizing.

Although I was a social worker and had facilitated many caregiving groups, being a primary caregiver was a new experience for me and I needed and used every support I could to help me through that time. The anguish is part of the process for all of us, the way grief and change can affect everyone. During that time, I realized I had to take care of myself as well as care for my husband.

Taking care can mean being mindful, or being alert, or having responsibility for or watching over. Some have used the term caretaking. I prefer caregiving since we are giving care. However, it is equally important that we take care of ourselves and are mindful of our actions both in caring for ourselves and others. Jim Austin, a dear friend of mine, said, "Taking care is an important part of everything we do. Without mindfulness our actions are often confused and/or misdirected. Without taking care of ourselves we have less ability to care for others...I believe that a care partnership would be empowering and very beneficial to both the process and the outcome of caring" when the care recipient is able to participate.

This book provides tools and techniques that I, as well as others, have used to care for ourselves and to make us more mindful as caregivers. I hope you will find them helpful in your caregiving journey. There is no specific way to use this book. Use it how it best works for you, whether you read it from cover to cover or look at the table of contents and read the chapters that seem pertinent to your situation.

The book is intended to help new caregivers caring for people with many different diagnoses. What is effective and fitting for one may not be for someone else. Use what resonates with your life style, your needs and those for whom you are caring.

The following provides an overview of the chapters:

- **Chapter 1 – Oh, No! Oh My God!** – is about how we integrate the change of circumstances into our lives. It provides examples of the emotions you may go through and reviews the five stages of grieving and dying as talked about by Dr. Elizabeth Kubler-Ross. I hope that once you realize that what you are going through is normal and that there is no right way to be a caregiver, it will enable you to manage more effectively.

- **Chapter 2 – Your Resource Manual.** It is vital that you know what the doctor(s) said and understand the implications. This chapter provides an organized method to keep critical information. This is especially important if a number of doctors and/or hospitals are involved. I recommend you keep at least a record of the basic facts.

- **Chapter 3 – Taking Care of Ourselves** offers some helpful strategies. If we do not take care of ourselves, it may be more challenging for us to care for our loved one. It is like the advice the flight attendants give you before takeoff. "Place the oxygen first over your own nose and mouth before placing it over your child's."

- **Chapter 4 – Knowledge is Power.** A short reminder that the more you know about the particular issue you and your loved one are dealing with, the better decisions you can make, care you can provide, understanding you and your loved one can have when something is not going as you expected.

- **Chapter 5 – Let Me Know if There is Anything I Can Do for You.** How often do we hear this from friends, neighbors, colleagues at work, parishioners from our place of worship? We nod in response, feeling overwhelmed yet at a loss to respond. Ways people can help are suggested. Frequently, receiving assistance is a gift not only for the receiver but also for the giver.

- **Chapter 6 – Finances and Legal Matters.** This chapter is a must read if the loved one is oriented, able to make decisions and the prognosis is poor. If you are unaware of what legal and financial papers are needed, this chapter will provide an overview for you. It includes an overview of living wills, durable power attorneys for health care which are important for all adults to have in place. Caregivers need them as well as care recipients.

- **Chapter 7 – Beyond Acceptance.** This is for those for whom spirituality is an important component in their lives. It provides a way to help you accept your loved one's death, if necessary.
- **Glossary.** This is to help with some of the terminology.
- **Appendix.** This provides some additional resources that may be helpful.
- **Guided Imagery.** This provides a sample of some guided imagery that you can record yourself and use to help relieve stress. Guided imagery is a method that focuses your imagination and your senses to decrease stress and increase a sense of well-being. Athletes have used it for years to improve performance and some cancer survivors say it contributed to their survival.

CHAPTER 1

OH NO! OH MY GOD!

Caregiving is tough. It tests the limits of human endurance - physically, emotionally, spiritually and for many, financially. Caregiving can be all consuming - occupying caregivers twenty-four hours a day, seven days a week. Handling the emotions can be as challenging as any other aspect. Many go through a wide spectrum of feelings not unlike those described by Dr. Elisabeth Kubler-Ross in her book, *Death and Dying*. Denial, depression, bargaining, anger and acceptance are all ways of coping. Some reach acceptance as she suggests; for others, the journey continues to be a formidable panoply of conflicting sensations; still others can get stuck in one place, perhaps denial or depression.

Everyone's path is unique because relationships differ, experiences are distinct and there are many diverse diagnoses and prognoses with which to cope. For some, it may be a gradual realization that something is wrong, or it can be a lightning strike. Mine began the day after my husband Bob had an MRI of his brain. I was checking the messages in my office when I heard his voice say, "It's a melanoma. We have an appointment at noon with our doctor and she wants you there. She's set up an appointment with an oncologist."

My journey begins

By the time I listened to my voice mail at work, I had already been through denial. (Cell phones were not as common then and I worked in a hospital where they are often not permitted.) When bob initially complained he was having trouble finding words, I thought it was due to stress because we were moving. I gradually realized something was wrong, yet never imagined it would be a brain tumor. When I received that incredible message, I thought, "Oh, no! Oh, my God!" and collapsed in my chair. I sat there stunned unable to process for some time. He was my touchstone for years so my next thought was that I needed to talk with him to find out how he was doing. I tried to reach him both at home and at work, but I could not locate him. I was glad I would see him soon so I could put my arms around him wanting to protect him from the dread disease growing in his brain and to reassure myself.

Denial is the firewall of the mind and can deceive the caregiver about the disease and how the care recipient will be affected by it. "I know my spouse is going to get better."

For a long time, I was angry because Bob had left a message and not spoken to me directly. On reflection, I realized that it was a small thing, a manageable focus, whereas the cancer and the idea that Bob might die were too devastating to handle. Instead, I displaced my anger onto Bob and what he had done. Being mad at him was easier for me than being angry at a disease. It never occurred to me that I was angry in order to cope or that it was part of the process. One day, months later, Bob said, "I did the best I could." I knew then I had to work through the anger and let it go

As was true in my case, the anger and frustration about the illness and its effects are often taken out on the care recipient or other family members. "If she asks me that question one more time, I'll scream."

because of the hurt I was causing him. We needed to stick together to get through this ordeal. So, I meditated, visualized releasing the anger, wrote an imaginary letter to him that I burned, cried, took long walks and talked to friends. Eventually, I moved on.

Most of the time, I alternated between numbness and depression. I couldn't imagine life without Bob. Relief came when my friend, Sophia, said with total disbelief in her voice, "You don't think he's going to die, do you?" I was so taken aback by her instant and positive response that I remained silent. The fact that someone who had an understanding of the disease believed that Bob was going to be okay gave me hope.

It helped to lift some of my depression. Prior to speaking with her, I would wake up about three in the morning and sob quietly into the pillow so that I wouldn't disturb Bob. Then, I'd fall back to sleep around five thirty, and have to get up at six thirty to get ready for work. I never seemed to get a restful sleep.

After the tumor was removed, Bob received whole brain radiation. This weakened his immune system and he went through bouts of other illnesses including pneumonia, pleurisy, and Bell's palsy. He was very weak and also required surgery for a double hernia. The friend we were living with felt that we had overstayed our welcome and asked us to move. Most apartments we looked at had over one hundred applicants. We were looking for a home that would be on one floor because I wasn't sure how his illness would play out in the coming years and wanted to be sure I could care

Often caregivers sleep poorly because so many things can happen to the care receiver while they are sleeping or because they are worried, anxious or depressed. Much of the time is spent with an ear open for anything that might be amiss. This is especially true if the care recipient is apt to wander or fall.

for him. Finally, after looking for two straight weeks we found an apartment that had two floors but Bob hadn't had his hernia surgery and was still very weak. We decided we could squeeze into the bottom floor and I would use the upstairs as a dressing room. The propane man who came to change the gas over to our name refused to turn it on because our bed was too close and we were unable to get it to the up-stairs. A friend lent us a space heater but that was also a problem. This was a very challenging time for us and particularly difficult for me as a caregiver.

Eventually we bought some land to build a house on. We wanted to show Bob's daughters where it was. They came to visit on a busy racing weekend so the bed and breakfast which was less than a mile from our new property was filled. We booked another. It was still quite obvious that Bob had been very ill. During a conversation with the proprietress of the bed and breakfast who had a scar running down the side of her face, I learned that she had been an oncology nurse so I said that Bob was recovering from a metastatic melanoma to the brain. She said, "That's what I had… a melanoma." She proceeded to relate her story which actually had occurred many years before when she was going to college. She now had children college age. I believed that it was no coincidence that we were brought together since it gave both Bob and myself hope that you can survive melanoma. Hope is so important to survival and to dealing with the stress of the illness.

Disability strikes

After the first year of acute care, Bob was much better. He had gone back to work and I thought the spread of the cancer was the only thing I needed to be concerned about. But almost two years after his surgery, Bob had a seizure, not the kind we traditionally think of when we talk about seizures. He didn't lose consciousness. He was at a

Dunkin Donuts on the way to a meeting. After getting his coffee and returning to the car, he couldn't figure out how to start the engine. He asked a woman who was passing by if she could start it. She did and he drove to the meeting. While there, Bob, a normally phenomenal note taker, could not write so that it made sense. He asked a retired doctor at the meeting if he should be concerned. The doctor told Bob that he should see a physician immediately.

Instead of going to his primary care physician in that same town, he drove a half an hour to see his neurosurgeon, Dr. P. By the time Bob reached the Dr. P's office, he was able to write without difficulty. Dr. P. was not there but was across town performing surgery. He was contacted and advised Bob that he was having a seizure and called in a prescription of dilantin, a common seizure medication.

I came home and heard a message from a neurologist's office indicating that Bob had an appointment the next day. What was that about? I thought they had dialed the wrong number. I wished they had dialed the wrong number.

After that, Bob's short term memory diminished, his capacity to think deteriorated, and his balance became impaired. All of these functions vacillated from pretty good to very awful in a jagged course such that hope sprang up only to be smashed to the ground.

Because of this up and down existence, I never knew how to answer , "How's Bob?" I didn't want to go into a long explanation. If he was having a good day, I was concerned if I said he was good that if something happened to him, people might think I misled them or that I was in denial or that I didn't want to share how he really was with them or any other number of thoughts. If he was having a bad day, I didn't want people to think every day is bad. It was difficult to know how to answer since how he was was often a moment by moment, day by day existence. I knew they were asking because they were concerned. Yet, I also didn't want them to think that my life was that hard.

Bob even on his most challenging days was still good company. We continued to share laughter. His easy going personality, natural empathy and willingness to do his part did not change. He thought of ways to give to others. Once he had bought this hand-made "tree" at a yard sale. To say I thought it was ugly and had no purpose would be an understatement. Finally we put it in our own yard sale but had no takers. While visiting a store, he noticed that part of their decoration was very similar to his "tree." He packed it up and took it over to the proprietor. With tears in his eyes, he recounted how touched and amazed she was to receive a smaller version of part of her store decoration.

In spite of his confusion and memory problems, he continued to be a political junky and took some adult education courses. I never knew how he did in the courses because he complained about not remembering what he read and often read the material two or three times in an effort to retain the information. I felt as long as they didn't kick him out of the class it was good for him to have the socialization and particularly in areas in which he remained interested.

I learned to focus on the positives, what worked for us and for him, rather than what didn't, what he could no longer do. I needed to remember and adjust to what he could no longer do. Bob could still do many tasks around the home providing I left him a reminder. I wrote down the steps for complicated chores.

One morning I asked him to mulch an area of the garden. The job required that he pull weeds around the good plants, put down newspapers where there were no seeds or plants, and then place mulch on all of the newspapers and around the good plants. When I came home I discovered that he had spread mulch everywhere including over the seeded area and over the iris rhizomes. I started to get upset at him for not doing it as I had asked him when I realized that I had not written down the directions. I said, "I'm sorry I forgot that you forget." This moment not only served to remind me of his disability but we were able to have a good laugh. And keeping our sense of humor has helped us both immeasurably.

I needed to remember that he was only trying to help me and was doing the best he could. I tried to keep that as my focus.

As time progressed and Bob continued to deteriorate, it became more difficult. I arranged for Meals-on-Wheels (which his brother and sister-in-law graciously offered to pay for) and for a cleaning woman to come in once a week. Ironically, it was a woman that had employed him for a short while to help her out on one of her jobs. When I saw her, I said, "I need help." She responded by saying she had known that when she saw my face. I also started to have friends stop in "when they were in the neighborhood." I knew that if he thought they were coming to check up on him that he wouldn't think he needed it but Bob had been very social. Yet the skills that had seemed so routine for him began to be a struggle. The gregarious man who would have talked with everyone on the beach by the end of the walk found it difficult to know what to say and it bothered him that he didn't always remember who they were or what he ought to know about them. When he had his memory, he could carry this kind of lapse off without anyone knowing but when he became more impaired he didn't like it showing.

Part of the strain I was under was my realization that Bob was deteriorating and that my caregiving role would increase until Bob died. I needed to come to grips with the idea of his dying. I was still not ready for that. When he was somewhat stable, I felt as though we had been given a new life. I hoped that our life together could return as it once was.

It never can. I recognized that life is a never-ending flow until we die and we don't get to repeat our favorite parts.

Bob's death had simply been deferred. I was still aware of the possible reoccurrence of the disease and how the side effects from his treatment would continue to affect our lives. When I thought about it, fear would hold me in its clutches – fear of his passing, fear of being alone, the pain of mourning.

I have meditated for nearly 40 years and felt I had to use that skill to accept his passing before the actual fact. I had accepted his illness because that was no longer an imminent threat, but I realized that the grim reaper was still present. He had only taken a holiday. I had to free Bob and do so with love. That didn't mean that he would die because I was ready, but that when he died, he would be able to do so without guilt or remorse, feeling only my love. It would be my greatest gift to him. I wasn't ready to do it with joy, and wasn't sure I would ever be able to, but I knew I needed to do it with love, not fear. This was such a challenge!

It is like the story of the little boy and his mother who were walking along the beach. The little boy asked his mother what love was like. She bent down and picked up some sand and squeezed it through her hand. "Notice, how when I hold on so tight the sand slips through my hand." Then she scooped up another handful of sand and just held it. "Notice this time how I am just holding the sand and it stays with me." Like the woman, I had to be able to hold Bob in my hand (and my heart) and just allow him to be, the hardest task to which I've ever committed. However, focusing on the joy, the love and the history we shared, helped me maintain my commitment.

The death watch

Bob began to have more falls and other accidents. He became very ill; it was unclear how he survived. Somehow beyond all reasonable belief, he got better. During his last hospitalization, the doctors were unable to find anything to help. Bob couldn't find words although he understood what was said to him. His walking was impaired; he seemed unable to move his feet and he couldn't maintain his balance. Since he seemed to improve during the day, the doctors thought he might be having sub clinical seizures (since he had had them in the past) but constant EEGs (encephalograms – used to check on brain waves) disproved that. MRIs and spinal tap found no cause. They reduced his seizure medication temporarily to see if that changed his brain waves; it did not. The doctors said it was a delayed reaction to the whole brain radiation. Somehow he got better. No one knew how or why; sometimes he was better and other times, awful.

His brother, Larry, who had Parkinson's became extremely ill and we were told that his time was near. Bob wanted to go see him in Pennsylvania but then when I advised him that he would not be able to drive he subtly changed his mind. Only later when he said he would go to the funeral when Larry died did I realize Bob had changed his mind so I wouldn't have to do all of the driving. It made no sense to me to go after Larry's death.

I packed us up to undertake the 8-9 hour drive to see his brother. I included Bob's living will, DPOA (Durable Power of Attorney) for healthcare, his medication sheet, extra medication and anything else that would be required if he got sick either enroute or while we were visiting. Amazingly, yet like many others that I have seen, Bob was better than he had been for a long time. He could talk although afterwards I realized that he had limited his conversation. He used his walker with no problems. He was able to see his brother and his sister who came up from Florida while we were there.

The day before we left he started to sleep a lot again. By the time we stopped for lunch he could not order and had difficulty using his walker. Once home he was too impaired to leave alone so I needed to take time off until I found someone to stay with him. I found someone who could come in for a few hours while I was at work. I believed that if he stayed at that level of care I could finish out the school year where I worked and then provide full time care until he passed away.

By using the process in the last chapter, I had reached the point where it was okay with me if he died. What he was going through was too difficult to watch. The kind, gentle, articulate man I married struggled with being alive.

On Friday May 30, 2008, Bob's nephew called to let us know that his father had passed away during the night. Bob was visibly shaken. He had said on the trip down to visit Larry that Bob had thought he would die first.

Then Sunday night Bob had difficulty moving his right arm. When he woke in the night to go to the bathroom, he could no longer move his right leg. By morning, he couldn't move his right arm, his right or left legs. I called his primary care physician and asked for an order for hospice. I also tried to get him admitted to the local hospice house but they did not have any openings and since he was not "actively dying" there would be a daily charge until he was in that stage. His neurologist called wanting to know why I didn't bring him in; he suggested they might be able to do something for him. I believed that since they had been unable to

There are two stages, the pre-active and the active stage of dying. In the pre-active stage, the person often has increased agitation and irritability, decreased intake of food and liquids, states that he or she is dying, requests family visits to settle "unfinished business, often reports seeing loved ones who have died before, and has increased swelling of the extremities of the body or the body in general. Generally in the active stage the person has stopped eating, often stops breathing for long periods of time, can be non-responsive and cold to the touch. For more information, see http://www.hospicepatients.org/hospic60.html

do anything for him the previous visit and the symptoms were similar, that the doctors would probably be unable to do anything this time either. Bob would certainly prefer to be at home to being in the hospital. The orders for hospice were delayed so I called to push the issue. Initially they told me they would not be out until Wednesday. I advised them that Bob had not voided from the night before. Immediately a social worker was dispatched to admit him to hospice and a nurse to catheterize him.

I also called our daughters to let them know the situation. The older one, Margaret, came to help me take care of him. It is no exaggeration to say that I couldn't have done it without her. I do not understand how people can care for others without assistance, particularly if the care recipients cannot turn themselves and are heavy. Turning Bob – which was required regularly – felt like moving a whale. He got so he could no longer swallow his medications or food. Since his seizure medication was discontinued, he started having convulsive seizures. Medication was administered for comfort – either through suppositories or by being absorbed in the mouth. Since he couldn't swallow, we found it best to rub it on the inside of his cheeks and mouth where it was absorbed by the body.

Although it took two of us to turn him, we tried to alternate times so that we could each get some rest. The necessity to give him his medication every two hours meant that two totally exhausted people became more exhausted. Somehow we did what we had to do. We were trapped in the house, our daughter more than myself because I had to run some errands. She tried going for walks but it was in the middle of black fly season in New Hampshire and they were voracious in attacking her. (Our daughter has always lived in the city so she has never needed or learned to drive.)

In the middle of all of this, our dog, Maggie, developed a cancer that was eating away at the bone in her leg. When she would not eat her treat I knew that she was in pain and I couldn't wait for the leg to fracture to ease her way. A friend agreed to take Maggie and me to the vet to put her to sleep.

About three days before Bob died, I had talked to a friend who mentioned that the hearing sense goes last and it might be helpful to play music or read to him. We began playing some music that he loved and some of the songs that he planned for his memorial service. He became very alert and at one point tried to talk which he hadn't tried in over a week. Only towards the end of the day did I realize that he might be able to blink in response to questions. I had him blink once for "yes" and twice for "no." I regret that I had not realized he could do that earlier in the day. That was the last day there was any communication from him.

It is very common for people who are dying to become alert and even more functional two to three days before they die. Although it did not give me hope, often families believe their loved one is getting better only to be severely disappointed when it is only temporary.

Bob had made arrangements for his body to be donated to Dartmouth Medical School so when it was clear that he was going to die, I called them to ascertain the proper procedure. The woman I spoke with asked some questions and reiterated that acceptance is not a sure thing and I should have alternate plans. Bob had made other plans but I opted for a provider who was closer. When Bob died, the school was not accepting bodies that day so I had to use the substitute plans with a local funeral home. I was glad I had made arrangements before he died. Some people make arrangements and pay for the funeral as part of their estate planning (wills, trusts, living wills, etc.)

When he died, I was both relieved and heartbroken. He had done a great deal of the legwork for his service and I only had to implement it. I had tried to urge our daughters to select prints for us to make a collage of his life but in the end, I did it. In a way, it served as a release as I relived his life and the part of it that I had shared. He was an amazing man, a thoughtful, kind, intelligent, gregarious soul whom I will miss dearly.

Friends and family have been incredibly supportive. A co-worker whose husband had died of cancer a couple of years before Bob died gave me this beautiful package of goodies. It included some poems that she liked and a Comfort Basket, developed by Anne Black, Ph.D. and contains concrete tools to help you grieve and care for your-self. One that I particularly liked was "A Letter to Your Loved One" with instructions not to rush the writing of this letter.

Comfort Baskets may be ordered through www.comfortbaskets.com, although my friend got mine at a local florist shop.

Grieving is different for everyone depending on family history, culture, relationship, suddenness of the death, age of the person who died and of the mourner. I find it is the unexpected moments, the waves that come crashing out of nowhere that are the hardest. I have a sensitive nose and to me, Bob always had a unique smell. In fact, when he was alive, I had tried to wash it out of his pillows. I assumed it would always be there since I had never been able to totally get rid of it. But shortly after he died I went to his pillow to inhale his smell, to feel a connection with him. There was no smell. I wept that I couldn't find it. About a month later I was about to throw out his hair brush when I decided to smell it. There it was so I kept the brush – at least for now.

There is a lot I need to do and some details I have to wait to carry out. I've done most of the paperwork and there is a lot of paperwork. I didn't have to go through Probate but I still needed to change our bank accounts, car insurance, etc. I haven't picked up his ashes. I haven't gone through all of his clothing. I have tried to reorganize my life and house and eventually, that will have to include both. I am fortunate to have done a lot of my grieving during the past year and while writing this book. I get annoyed when people ask me how I am and I say I'm good and they don't believe me. It doesn't mean I'm always good; it means at that moment I'm good. I feel that some people would be happier if I were not doing well. I am trying to live in the moment. Like all of life, sometimes it's good and sometimes it's not.

Experiencing and learning to cope with a wide range of emotions is part of the caregiving and grieving process. The history and relationship with the care recipient, the caregiver's beliefs, the daily stressors, the severity of the diagnosis, the physical demands of caregiving, the coping skills of the caregiver all affect the caregiver's emotional experience. Each caregiver's reaction is unique, yet all caregivers deal with stress and a wide range of feelings. Following are some condensed examples from friends, family members, and clients.

Questioning your faith & beliefs

Jeannette was catapulted into caregiving when her mother had a stroke and became partially paralyzed. Her mother, Bernadette, had gone for rehabilitation and learned how to care for herself with her new limitations. By the time she left the facility, Bernadette was able to load the dishwasher, prepare some meals, and clean and dress herself. The social worker at the facility had arranged for meals-on-wheels to be delivered and provided a referral for a home health aide to do some shopping and cleaning. One day Jeannette stopped by unannounced and found her mother still in her nightgown. Even in the nursing home, Bernadette had gotten dressed every morning and applied her make-up. Jeannette noticed stacks and stacks of dirty dishes in the sink. Bernadette couldn't remember if she had eaten breakfast or lunch. Jeannette realized her mother was going to need more care and attention than she had been receiving.

Jeannette was already weighed down with caring for her own family, and the idea of assuming responsibility for her mother was unthinkable. She asked her sister, Barbara, for help but she lived too far away and was not inclined to get involved. Jeanette tried adding a stop on the way home from work, but that did not provide sufficient care for her mother. Taking her into their home wasn't an option because there was no room. Bernadette refused to consider an assisted living facility, and said that if Jeannette thought there was a problem, then she could continue to stop by enroute home from work. Jeannette found herself losing patience with everyone: her husband, her mother, her children, and even her co-workers.

Jeannette had always had a deep faith in God, but when her mother began to have these difficulties, she began to question her beliefs. She wondered, "Why me? What did I do to deserve this?" She felt she had tried to lead a good life. She knew that she was far from perfect, but she didn't think either she or her mother had done anything to warrant this fate. She asked God to make her mother better. When this didn't work, she promised God that she would be more generous to the less fortunate and be faithful to her husband, not only in deed, but in thought. Perhaps that was where she had gone astray. None of it seemed to be successful. Her mother still couldn't seem to function as well as she had. Jeannette's bargaining did not work.

Finally, she acknowledged to herself that she would have to do something she had always vowed she wouldn't: put her mother in a nursing home over her mother's objections. However, she learned that her mother did not yet meet the criteria for nursing home care and was pleased to discover that her father had paid for long term care insurance. Bernadette, in spite of her confusion, had continued to pay the premiums. Soon, Jeannette was able to find an appropriate facility near her home.

To Bernadette's surprise, she enjoyed being cared for and talking with the other residents. Indeed, she seemed to improve with the attention and stimulation provided. Consistent mealtimes, a smooth routine, and companionship helped her regain her emotional balance. Her confusion decreased, her memory returned to where it had been when she left the rehabilitation center, and she was happier. Like many older people, she had been more depressed than demented. Jeannette took over paying the bills for Bernadette so she had no responsibilities. And, because she lived closer to Jeannette, they actually saw each other more often than before.

Jeannette believed a miracle had occurred. She had her mother back. Maybe God was listening! She got down on her knees and prayed with joy, thankfulness and tears.

Battling depression

When Sydney's wife, Anna, was initially diagnosed with COPD (chronic obstructive pulmonary disease – chronic bronchitis and/or emphysema), it didn't seem like a major problem. Her doctor explained that Anna's cabaret singing when she was in her twenties and thirties exposed her to second-hand smoke, the culprit in Anna's disease. Now in her fifties, Anna's need for oxygen increased and her ability to complete simple household tasks decreased, Sydney finally understood that Anna would not get better and that he would outlive her. He felt as though someone had punched him in the stomach. He had never before thought about losing her or living life without her. Or if he had, it would be in the distant future when they were both very old.

Subsequent to this realization, he found he couldn't concentrate or focus on his normal outlets of television or reading. They were too challenging. All he was able to do was pace or do something that required activity. He could not abide any sedentary pursuits. When he tried to relax, he felt like the world was closing in. When he wasn't pacing, he was eating. He had difficulty sleeping, often walking up and down the upstairs hall. He was exhausted all the time. Although he had always found humor in unusual situations, nothing was funny. He tried to joke with his wife to cheer her up and the jokes seemed to fall flat.

During moments of anguish, he would rail against his wife's early career even though that was how he had met her. After months of feeling this desolation, Sydney, in desperation, asked his doctor for some sleeping pills. As a result of the ensuing discussion, his doctor recognized Sydney's symptoms as depression and offered him an anti-depressant. The anti-depressant allowed Sydney to begin to cope with the challenges of caring for his wife.

He continued to work, deciding that he would do so until Anna could no longer manage with the supports he put in place. Sydney found that focusing on his job helped distract him from the immediate day-to-day stressors of caring for a dying wife. It normalized the situation since Anna had always

Although all caregivers feel depressed and sad at some time, it is important to distinguish between normal sadness or the blues and clinical depression. A majority of caregivers do experience clinical depression. For those caring for people with dementia the percentage is higher. The signs of clinical depression include depressed mood, lack of interest in normal activities, significant weight loss or gain, difficulty sleeping or sleeping a lot, lack of energy, restlessness or a feeling of being slowed down, feeling worthless or excessively guilty, inability to think or concentrate, or thought of suicide. If you have five or more of these over a two-week period, you may have clinical depression and should see your primary care physician or a psychiatrist.

www.depression-screening.org offers not only a self-screener but video testimonials and additional information on depression. If you feel you want to take your life, call 911 or go immediately to an emergency room.

been a stay-at-home wife. Anna was glad that he kept working because she would have felt guilty about him leaving his job. Although Anna missed him, she slept or rested most of the time, so it was not an issue. She had worried that he might lose his job if he didn't continue to work. And she found that she didn't have to try to be at her best all the time.

Confronting guilt

While caring for her mother, Martha reported feeling guilty just going to the mailbox, or picking up a video, or performing any other short errand that meant she would not be instantly available. Martha felt that it wasn't rational. Another part of her mind kept telling her that she should be happy to care for her mother, that she was being an ungrateful daughter, that she shouldn't be angry with her mother because her mother couldn't help it. And she had promised her father when he died that she would take care of her mother.

Yet clearly, she needed to be able to run errands. Finally, she got a cell phone with a walkie-talkie so her mother could call her if there was an emergency. Initially, her mother used it all the time Martha was away, which irritated her because she now had no privacy, no time of her own, not even the time it took to walk down the driveway to the mailbox. Gradually, the novelty wore off for her mother and Martha figured out that the best time to do errands was when her mother was watching her favorite TV shows. By knowing that her mother could reach her if there was a real emergency, she felt at ease running the needed errands.

Many people make bedside promises to one parent to care for the other parent when the latter parent is widowed. As much as we want to honor our promises and feel guilty when we don't, most of us do not understand how draining the job of caregiving can be. It is not unusual for caregivers to still experience awakening at night or being jittery long after the care recipient is no longer in the household.

Frustration in dealing with denial and military culture

When James was called to serve in Iraq as part of the Army National Guard, neither he nor his wife envisioned the marked changes that would occur in their lives when he returned. Shanja became one of the silent and unrecognized caregivers of soldiers returning from combat, not with physical injuries but with injuries to their psyche.

When James left for Iraq, Shanja went back to work full time and placed JJ, their six month old son, in day care. She didn't particularly want to but financially they now needed the extra income since James' regular income was no longer coming in. They missed each other dreadfully and found ways to communicate on-line, by phone and text messages. It was very hard for Shanja because, of course, as soon as James left, there was a problem with the sink leaking. Normally, James would simply have fixed the problem or if he couldn't, he would have

Because mental health issues are often not as obvious as physical ones, many underestimate the stress that partners and caregivers experience and the amount of caregiving required. However, just as physical issues vary greatly from individual to individual so do mental issues. For example, some with diabetes manage their illness with exercise and diet; others need insulin and have difficulty with their illness and its side effects. There are also many functional people with mental illnesses and many who cannot function.

called one of his buddies to come help him. Most of his buddies had gone with him so Shanja now had to find a plumber and arrange for someone to be there when he came. Then one morning she woke up and the house was cold. After checking to make sure JJ wasn't too cold and had enough blankets, she went to the basement and discovered that although there was oil, the furnace was not working. She was able to resolve this but it seemed as though James' leaving had created more trauma than just his departure. Although Shanja had initially been intimidated by the challenges, over time she began to be more confident in her skills to handle whatever the situation offered. She became more self-assured at work and increased her job skills such that she was offered and accepted a promotion. She was delighted not only with the promotion and the extra money but also was proud of her ability to handle everything that had happened since James was in Iraq.

JJ and she bonded because on the weekends he had her total attention. Time that might have been spent with both of his parents or shared with them now was focused entirely on him.

Meanwhile, James was undergoing his own culture shock in Iraq, the realities of combat, the change in climate, and the challenges of dealing with people who do not speak your language and whose language you do not understand. James also witnessed one of his best friends losing a leg.

About two days before James was to return, he got some shrapnel in his legs. He was treated but the injuries, although bothersome, were not considered significant so he was only slightly delayed in getting home.

But things were different. JJ did not recognize him and was intimidated by his Dad. Shanja, although delighted to see him, realized shortly after he was home that James had changed substantially too. She was a light sleeper so the first night that James woke up, sitting bolt upright in the bed, she woke up also. Shanja asked what was wrong but James said it was nothing and told her to go back to sleep. This soon became a pattern. James would jump when Shanja came up behind him to put her arms around him. Finally, he asked her not to surprise him anymore. James who had always been very easy going seemed to be more irritable. He didn't want to talk about his experience in Iraq, simply stating that it was over now and time for them to move on with their own lives. James found that tasks that he had always done were now capably handled by Shanja and not necessarily the way he had always carried them out.

Their adjustment to each other was stressful. James who had been affectionate and loving seemed to have more difficulty talking about and demonstrating his feelings. His return to work was not smooth either. He seemed to have trouble focusing on the task at hand, often being distracted, but not willing to discuss it. Prior to serving in the war, James had a good relationship with his manager, but his inability to concentrate and complete his work in a timely fashion and his reluctance to talk about it put a strain on their relationship.

One day, Shanja was talking with her grandfather who had served in World War II. She confided in him about what James was going through but her grandfather was not helpful. He said, "Oh, sounds like he's going through a little bit of shell shock. It will soon pass ... Besides, you don't want him getting treated for anything like that, it will ruin his chances of being able to retire with the Army National Guard. Just give him time."

However, armed with this information, Shanja went online to learn more. In the process she found information on PTSD (Post Traumatic Stress Disorder) and she began to compare James' behavior with the criteria for the syndrome. She

PTSD can occur when someone experiences a traumatic event that causes that person to feel intense fear, helplessness or horror. The event can include war, natural disasters, rape, abuse, serious accidents and captivity.

Veterans and their spouses can go to www.militarymentalhealth.org to take a screening to verify if the involved vet might have the symptoms of PTSD. Anyone may go to www.nami.org to find support and assistance. NAMI is the National Alliance for the Mentally Ill and provides support to families of mentally ill.

soon became convinced that it was a good possibility that James did have PTSD but when she mentioned it to him, he refused to discuss it, reiterated her grandfather's viewpoint about not being able to stay in the Guard, and asked her if she thought he was crazy.

As things continued to deteriorate in their relationship, Shanja became more desperate and was considering leaving James when she discovered she was pregnant again. She loved James but was having difficulty living with his sleeplessness, his irritability, the ongoing tension, his exaggerated response to nearly everything, his denial about there being a problem.

Finally she went on-line again to find out what benefits might be available to him because she felt his symptoms were a combat-related disorder and that he should be getting help through the Guard. Frightened lest she bring another child into this unhappy home and not wanting to be a single parent to two small children, she begged James to at least go talk to someone, if only to prove her wrong. Each time she suggested; he rejected and got angrier. She talked to his parents who likewise encouraged him to seek assistance.

James, of course, was feeling increased pressure at home and at work. The pressure seemed to have the opposite affect from that desired. The more pressure, the less willing he seemed to be to seek help.

Finally, Shanja could take no more and tearfully gave him an ultimatum as well as the information he needed to get assistance. It was only as she began to pack her things and those of the children that he realized she was serious and took steps to get help.

James was able to get services and found a psychotherapist who knew some of the more effective treatments for PTSD including EMDR (Eye Movement Desensitization and Reprocessing) and EFT (Emotional Freedom Techniques).

EMDR uses a very structured use of bi-lateral stimulation to the brain to reprocess the trauma. The bi-lateral stimulation can be through eye movement in which the client's eyes follow the fingers of the clinician or an eye bar, or through listening to sounds alternating between the left and right ears or through tapping on hands or knees or a combination of the above. EFT uses tapping on points used in acupuncture. Both are using bi-lateral stimulation to the brain. For more information, see the websites listed in the sidebar. Using these modalities in conjunction with normal psychotherapy, James has made substantial progress. However, it is unclear at this time what role he will have in the Guard, if any.

Patricia Resick of Boston University has developed Cognitive Processing Therapy (CPT) , a twelve session program that is also helping victims of PTSD.

For more information about EMDR and to find a clinician near you, go to www.EMDR.com. For EFT, go to www. eftuniverse.com.

Loss of dreams

Jared and Morgan were an ideal couple in their mid-twenties. They had everything going for them – popular, bright, incredibly attractive. They had unbelievably well paying jobs and had just purchased their first home, a fixer-upper. When renovated, their new home would be worth a fortune. In spite of them both working sixty-hour work weeks, this high-energy couple planned to do much of the work themselves – until Morgan was in an automobile accident that changed their lives. She sustained a serious spinal cord injury in addition to broken bones.

When Jared received the telephone call, he was sure there was a mistake and set off to the hospital determined to correct the error of identity. He was stunned when he walked into the Intensive Care Unit and saw her hooked up to machines. Feeling overwhelmed, distraught and confused, he couldn't seemed to make sense of it all. He could see her but a part of him still didn't believe it. He felt numb and had difficulty focusing. He spent the next three days in the hospital by her side with friends and family. Finally, her parents urged him to go home, get some rest and take care of himself.

Jared kept his employer up-to-date on Morgan's condition and although his manager was initially sympathetic, as time went on he began to insist on Jared's imminent return. Jared was torn; he felt an obligation to work and clearly one of them needed to be working but the love of his live was lying in a hospital bed and the resulting pain penetrated to the very depths of his being. He could not leave her. At other moments, he thought he was insane and should be doing his job. He tried to do some of his work on his laptop at the hospital and at home in the evenings but he was unable to focus. He resigned himself to the probable loss of his job and the house.

Then a friend reminded him of the family leave act. He called Human Resources and was indeed eligible. He would receive no pay but he would not lose his job and it would give them time and maybe the opportunity to figure out how disabled Morgan was. It was unclear when or if she would work again and they had purchased their home based on both of their incomes.

The person in Human Resources provided him with the telephone number of their Employee Assistance Program (EAP) and reminded him that the EAP could provide counseling, financial information and other helpful resources. When Jared called his EAP representative, she provided him with a number for a counselor who specialized in dealing with people who suffered from paralysis and their caregivers.

When Morgan was well enough to talk, she suggested that he might want to divorce her. She told him that she didn't want to be a burden to him. He was shocked by her offer and couldn't imagine life without her regardless of her condition. They decided to explore counseling with the specialist after her rehabilitation.

Morgan went for rehabilitation and some feeling did come back but insurance only pays for so much rehabilitation. They discussed options. Jared investigated making their fixer-upper accessible for Morgan's needs but the cost was prohibitive. The physical and occupational therapists did an assessment of their home and discouraged them from putting any work into the house.

The Family & Medical Leave Act of 1993 permits up to 12 weeks of unpaid leave for eligible employees and continued medical coverage (paid for by the employee). Companies that have less than 50 employees do not have to offer this.

Jared was stretched. He had returned to work when Morgan went to the rehab. He got up at 5 in the morning, ate a small breakfast, drove an hour to work, performed his job duties until 6 or later at night and then visited Morgan at the rehab, went home, made his dinner, and fell into bed exhausted. He didn't think he could do anymore. Weekends, he tried to catch up at home on household details like bills, laundry, groceries, etc. and still visited his beautiful lady for most of Saturday and Sunday.

He was visiting her on a Sunday when the question of what they were going to do was brought up. He knew, had always known in some part of his being, that they would never return to their new home together. The visits by the therapists had confirmed that but discussing it made it real for both of them. They wept in each other's arms. Morgan decided that she could not even go back and look at the house. They agreed to explore other options. Jared was the only one capable of carrying out all of the details necessary to put their home on the market, pack, and find new housing.

He started packing the next day before he came to visit her. After roaming from room to room, having difficulty concentrating and starting on one area, Jared nearly broke his hand while he repeatedly rammed it into the wall. He knew he couldn't pack and called his parents. They offered to pay a portion of the cost to have the home moved by professionals. He felt he was a coward but every dish, every garment, even the sports equipment he had tried to box up reminded him of his losses, their dreams, his remarkable wife who was now paralyzed. His inability to cope with carting up the home and all it represented changed him. Although he laughed and joked with his friends, it was a long time before he was able to visit their homes and see their children. He didn't begrudge them happiness. He just couldn't be reminded that he would never have that. Indeed a part of him was glad of the excuse of visiting Morgan and taking care of her that allowed him to avoid them.

Eventually they sold their dream home and moved into a condominium that had an elevator. Since they bought it during the building stages they were able to ensure that the doors and counters were wheelchair appropriate. But their dreams of children and travel to exotic and out-of-the-way places ended with the accident. Although Morgan was eventually able to return to work, she could no longer maintain the schedule that she had previously and Jared found it easier to help her with the areas of her care that required support than pay for someone else. They were on the fast track to monetary success, children and early retirement but their lives were changed instantaneously.

Sense of isolation

Sarah was George's second wife. They had both retired early and had made plans for a wonderful new life together. They bought a home out in the country so that they could observe the birds and other wildlife from their sun porch. Then, Sarah was diagnosed with a terminal illness.

Initially, the changes were subtle and they were able to maintain a comfortable lifestyle. But as the disease progressed, Sarah became an invalid and her sunny personality changed into that of a demanding shrew. The cost of the medications was consuming their retirement funds. The sanctuary in the woods became a prison. It was too far out for people to drop in routinely. When they did stop by, Sarah, like many ill people, seemed to call upon untold reserves and appear to be much better than she was. When their friends from the ski or book clubs called, their questions were always about Sarah. It seemed Sarah and her illness con-

Many very sick people somehow rally when non-caregivers are around or when visitors come. I had a schizophrenic patient who could dress herself and go to a job interview and always get the job. When I first brought her to the psychiatrist, she was so asymptomatic that he questioned if she had a mental illness.

sumed their lives. George thought he didn't count anymore because everyone always asked about Sarah - not about him and how he was doing. After all, she was the sick one.

George felt isolated. People did not appear to understand the difficulties he faced because Sarah always gave the impression that she wasn't that sick. He became so stressed while providing care for her needs and demands that he thought of leaving her, but he knew he wouldn't be able to live with himself if he did. In private, he asked her doctors about her life expectancy. He felt if he knew, he could pace himself; he could figure out if he would be able to care for her without collapsing himself. A member of their congregation asked him what he would do differently if he had this information. What would he change? George found he couldn't answer the questions, but somehow thinking about those questions helped him.

He began to attend a support group and arranged for Sarah's friends to come in and care for her daily to supplement the Visiting Nurses. These breaks helped him to manage, although it remained difficult.

Caring for someone who has changed

John didn't mind tending his wife Mina who had a form of dementia. At first, it wasn't the daily routine of caring and responding to the problems that was the challenge, but rather that the Mina he knew and loved had disappeared inside the body of someone who knew him but seemed only to tolerate his caregiving and presence. Mina would often look quizzically at him as if to say, "And who are you again?"

They had always been devoted to each other and he missed the Mina he knew, the one who laughed when he told a joke for the umpteenth time, the one who cuddled every night before they fell asleep, the one with whom he could share ideas. But most of all, he missed his best friend. It was the loss of the emotional connection that was so painful. He mourned his old relationship and tried to develop one with the new Mina. But the new Mina didn't have the shared history, the same knowing and understanding of who he was or what they had been through together.

The old Mina continued to disappear more and more until there was only the new Mina, the one that required almost total care, the one who had no sense of humor, the one who didn't see why she had to take a bath or why he couldn't feed her when he just had. As each part of the old Mina stopped working, John grieved its passing. With each new bewildering event, John felt a part of him and his relationship with the old Mina die.

Eventually the twenty-four hour a day, seven days a week care became overwhelming for John. His only break came when someone came in to care for her so he could get groceries. His health began to be affected by the constant caregiving. Against family members' objections, he placed Mina in a nursing home. It didn't seem to bother her because her behavior remained the same. He was initially overcome with guilt and questioned his decision. Part of him eventually realized it was another stage of the process and mourned their old life. When Mina finally died, he felt he had already grieved her passing and was quietly relieved.

Using determination

When Celia's husband broke his back in an accident at work, she insisted that he do as much for himself as he could in spite of the fact that he really wanted to be waited on. However, she was committed to her full-time job and now had sole responsibility for their children. Prior to the accident, Bryan had done most of the cooking so Celia had to take over that chore as well. Bryan's doctor wanted him to be active, providing he wore his brace, to help prevent him developing pneumonia. His doctor told him that it would take a while to heal but that it was good for him to walk. Due to the pain and his fear of further injury, Bryan resisted movement. Eventually, Celia and his doctors were able to coax Bryan to begin walking.

Celia continued to work and left simple food for Bryan to prepare for himself; gradually, he started to make his meals. As the pain decreased, he began to walk farther. The more he walked, the better he felt and the longer he walked. Despite most patients' objections, healing is aided by doing as much as possible for themselves. This was certainly true for Bryan, whose doctors were amazed at his progress.

Celia was able to focus on her job, caring for the children and coping with the additional chores and stress. One of the unanticipated stressors was that Bryan was now around all of the time. Celia hadn't realized how much she valued her own space. She created ways to be by herself, puttering around in her garden, going for short walks with the dog, hiding with a book in the family room, or playing her piano. She decided to learn the trumpet. She found if she really needed to be alone she just had to start practicing her trumpet and the family would find other places to be. Sometimes we need to be very resourceful to help us cope with the change in circumstance or our emotions and those of our family. She was glad and knew she was lucky when her caregiving days were over and Bryan was able to return to work.

Accepting a child's disability

Sam and Cindy had always wanted children so even though Cindy was in her late thirties when she became pregnant, they were cautiously optimistic. When Joshua was born they were ecstatic. Joshua was a very verbal child who easily found favor with all of their friends. When he started school he didn't make friends his own age as his parents had expected he would. But Sam and Cindy didn't worry about that. As far as they were concerned he was the perfect little boy, the child that made their life complete. In his early years the teachers commented about Joshua's poor social skills and his inability to understand basic social cues. Sam and Cindy attributed this to the fact that boys tend to develop more slowly than girls.

Joshua was their only child. Most of their friends were older and their children were not going through the same developmental stage as Joshua, so they could not compare Joshua with other children his age. By third grade when Joshua began to study more complicated mathematics, the teachers again reiterated their concerns. Now not only did Joshua lack social skills, have no class friends, have difficulty understanding math, he also seemed overly sensitive to sounds and was not very well coordinated. His primary teacher asked if Joshua collected anything. Of course, Sam and Cindy had always been delighted with Joshua's knowledge and interest in the Civil War and had encouraged his collection of books, facts, and posters about the subject. They acknowledged that when he started talking about it, Joshua seemed reluctant to stop, but they were privately pleased that their son could be so brilliant and informed in this area and already had him pegged as a future famous historian.

His teacher suggested that their son might have a Pervasive Developmental Disorder (whatever that was!) and that she would like to have him tested. Cindy and Sam could not believe it! What would the testing show? What did PDD mean? What did that have to do with anything? He didn't have friends because he was beyond them intellectually and knew words that others didn't understand. They were sure that was the situation and eventually, his social skills would catch up. For nearly six months the teacher worked to persuade Josh's parents that he should be evaluated. Finally, they agreed because he did appear to be having continued trouble with math.

When Cindy and Sam heard that the testing showed that Joshua had Asperger's Syndrome, they didn't understand or believe it and decided to have their own assessment done. After checking around, they went to a psychologist, Dr. O., who had a good reputation and was known to work with children with these diagnoses. Sam and Cindy were sure that since Dr. O. specialized in this area she would be able to see that Joshua was not like those other children. But Dr. O confirmed the results of the other testing and was able to explain the diagnosis in a way they were able to understand and accept.

Initially they were devastated. The night of the diagnosis they wept together. They couldn't believe their wonderful child had something wrong with him. Slowly as they learned and read more about the disorder they realized that at least it was a diagnosis that Joshua could live with and still be successful. Indeed, many famous people were alleged to have the disorder. To help learn social skills and to cope with his differences, Joshua went to Dr. O for therapy.

Gradually, Cindy and Sam realized it explained many of the questions they had had about Joshua which they had attributed to their own lack of knowledge about children. Because of his diagnosis and problems in math, the school district provided him assistance through special education. Cindy and Sam learned to use social stories to help him understand social situations. They became active in their local support group and the state organization. They learned to advocate for Joshua in school. He joined a club for Civil War buffs, a way for him to share his knowledge and develop friendships. Although Joshua continues to misunderstand some social situations, both he and the family continue to learn and make adjustments.

Grieving a child

My friend Susan's caregiving began when she realized that her son Harry wasn't just having headaches but difficulty with physical coordination. Harry had always loved sports, especially running and cross-country skiing and had recently taken up snow-boarding, his new joy. But Harry began to struggle doing maneuvers that had been routine for him. He would occasionally mention headaches but Susan suffered from headaches too, so she thought they were just a normal part of life.

When she saw him fight to maintain his balance, she took him to his doctor immediately. Initially she felt guilty that she hadn't taken his headaches more seriously. Then she wondered if the local doctors knew what they were doing. When Harry was finally referred to a specialist at a teaching hospital two hours away, his new doctor showed her pictures from his MRI and Susan knew her son would have an uphill battle. Because some of the treatment could alter his fertility, Harry's doctor asked if Harry would like to save some of his sperm before they began treatment. Harry was embarrassed and Susan was initially appalled. He declined.

Susan's anger consumed her. She was infuriated at God, whom she wasn't even sure she believed in, at her ex-husband for not being available, at her present husband for his lack of concern and his drinking, and at the doctor. She even got annoyed at her son, and then felt guilty because she knew he couldn't help it. And she was mad at herself - that was the worst of all. But she wanted him to put up more of a fight, she wanted Harry to win and it looked as though the cancer was winning. She didn't know how she would handle it if he died.

Compassionate Friends is a national organization dedicated to helping bereaved parents, grandparents and siblings toward the positive resolution of grief at losing a child regardless of age.
www.compassionatefriends.org or 1-877-969-0010 can assist families to find a local chapter.

Although Susan wasn't really a believer, in desperation she promised God if He would cure Harry she would dedicate her life to Him. But, her bargaining gained her nothing. The inexorable course of the cancer won, defeating her and her son. Susan became very depressed. She didn't see how she could go on; she didn't want to go on; she wanted to be with her son. Then there would be no more pain. She struggled with the pain for months. She had quit her job to care for Harry and now he was gone and she had nothing. She kicked her husband out and sank deeper into depression.

One day, a friend came by to see Susan and found her, disheveled and sobbing in the bedroom. Her face was blotchy; her eyes swollen. Clothes were strewn throughout the house. Susan hadn't eaten or bathed in days, the dishes were not done, the house was a wreck. Susan's friend got her up, fed her, ran her a bath, called her doctor and helped her clean her house. Gradually, with help, Susan got better. She started to participate in Compassionate Friends. She started to do activities to honor Harry's memory, establishing a fund at the college for athletic students whose families could not supply them with equipment. She's not sure she has reached total acceptance and is not sure there is such a thing, but she is closer and she is glad that Harry is not suffering anymore.

Coping with our emotions

Although the vignettes above each highlight one or two emotional responses, it is rarely as simple as that. The fear about the diagnosis and its real or imagined impact, the stress of caregiving, the amount of emotional support received, the extent the care recipient requires assistance with activities of daily living, the availability of supports and our ability to secure them, an individual's coping skills and family history, the care recipient's memory and judgment, and the caregiver's own health and age affect our emotions.

Emotions are signals to remind us that we are alive, that we have challenges to meet, and that we have joys, love, and pain to share. Sharing is a way of dealing with all of the emotions we go through during this period. I found my friends an incredible resource and support. Caregivers can be overwhelmed by the reactions, the additional and ongoing responsibilities, the communication needs, the stress. Sometimes it can all seem too much, especially if you are in a rural community or have few supports. Often caregivers feel isolated; that they need to carry this burden on their own. (See chapter 5, "Let Me Know If There Is Anything I Can Do" for ways others can help you.)

Stress can affect our ability to provide care and be effective in our own lives. Although Chapter 3, "Taking Care of Ourselves," offers a wide range of solutions to help deal with it, the following ideas can be used immediately.

Journaling, writing down our feelings, experiences and reflections, is a technique that many have used to help deal with the array of feelings we experience. It can put life in perspective, allowing feelings to surface rather than stuffing them down. It enables us to pass through the terror and come out on the other side. In such stressful times, I think of the story of Tamino and Pamina in Mozart's *The Magic Flute*. In order for them to enter the Temple of Light, they have to go through several ordeals. This reminds me that we too have to experience the pain before there is hope for release. Writing it down and keeping the record in its own book helps many to process the anguish.

Caregivers often find it difficult to get sufficient or good rest. When Bob was first sick I found it very challenging to get adequate sleep. I took every opportunity to relax, rest or sleep in. Otherwise I was concerned that I would burn out before his illness ran its course.

As I mentioned earlier, anger was part of the series of emotions I went through. Anger is very common and really is about our fears and our powerlessness. When we feel we have no control over the situation, anger and frustration are easier to cope with than the fear. Looking at the feelings, figuring out what we're covering up, can make it easier to manage.

One of the ways Bob and I consistently dealt with stress in our marriage was through laughter. Bob had a wonderful sense of humor which he was able to bring to most situations. Shortly after his surgery to remove the brain tumor, his mother died. His hair on one side of his head was still growing back after being shaved for surgery. During the reception after the funeral, one of the ladies in the church came up to me and asked if that was a new hairstyle Bob was sporting. This provided us a good laugh for a long time.

I encourage all caregivers to hold onto the humorous moments. They are gifts from God. Humor also helps us to heal and counteracts the effects of stress. Many times a painful incident when viewed later through the lens of time and distance can seem funny. These moments assist us to keep life in perspective.

Our viewpoint can change. Time continues to be a great healer. It is not that the pain goes away but that the intensity is eased. It can change the type of caring that we need to provide. The disease may have progressed, it may be cured or in remission, it may have become a chronic, managed disease.

Hope was another gift I received and helped to relieve the burden I was carrying. A friend suggested I was in denial. As far as I was concerned I had changed my focus from fear of his death to hope for his future. Since he was still with me nearly seven years later, my change of attitude enabled us to enjoy that time instead of focusing on the dread disease he had. I saw what time we did have together as a gift. For us, hope and humor were very important.

Whether you come to caregiving by choice or default or a combination, when possible, center your attention on any positives you can find, see the opportunity to be a caregiver as a gift, because caregiving may be the hardest task you have ever undertaken.

CHAPTER 2

YOUR RESOURCE MANUAL

When Bob was first diagnosed with a brain tumor, there was so much information I had to keep track of while I was still trying to adjust to the fact that he had cancer. My friend, Chris, whose husband, Ron, had survived cancer, suggested I get a notebook and keep track of appointments and questions. I call my variation a resource manual. By keeping it, I didn't have to worry about remembering everything. And, there sure was a lot of stuff going on in my head.

Because Bob's tumor was in the brain, it was vital for one of us to keep track of details and I found the resource manual invaluable. Bob also referred to it when he needed clarification for an upcoming test or a new prescription or the answer to a question he had asked before.

The stress of caregiving and the shock of the initial diagnosis affects our memory, making it difficult to remember important facts. By creating your own resource manual and bringing it with you to every medical appointment or event, you can maintain a record of each and information for when you have questions.

CREATING YOUR OWN

I used a two-inch D-ring binder with sections for easy additions and deletions as needed. I was surprised how fast this filled up, but you can of course start with a smaller size. You can create your own resource manual by using the following instructions (or you can download the pages from my website, www.joanperry.net). Another friend opted to use 3x5 cards that she could shuffle through as needed.

INSIDE COVER

On the inside cover of your binder, be sure to tape **a copy of your name and address and a copy of the patient's medical insurance.** (If you are concerned about identity theft, think of this as important as your wallet and remember to keep it with you at all times.) This provides a quick reference should you need it. If the manual gets misplaced, the information would enable someone to return it to you.

Because your manual is a resource for both everyday and emergencies, use the front of the binder for information about emergencies.

FIRST PAGE

A typed or printed **list of all of the patient's doctors**. This typed (or clearly printed) sheet should be placed in a clear plastic sleeve so you can access the appropriate doctor's number. Include the name of each doctor, his/her address and phone number, his/her specialty in both technical and lay terms, i.e. neurologist = brain/nerve/spinal doctor, oncologist = cancer doctor. This helps you begin to understand the medical terms and the roles each doctor plays in your particular patient's life, and is especially helpful if there are specialties within specialties.

SECOND PAGE

Although it may not be used in an urgent situation, **a list of organizations, addresses and telephone numbers** is important. This could include hospice, Visiting Nurse Associations (VNA), home health aides, religious affiliates, school numbers, those who may provide respite care for you, people who may be providing transportation when you are unavailable and/or companionship to the patient. It is also helpful to include the names of the individual providers. For example, if there is one particular nurse who comes regularly from the VNA, then include that information along with the company name.

BINDER SECTIONS
CALENDAR

The first actual section of the binder should be a calendar for appointments. This should include all appointments whether they are for doctors, dialysis, chemotherapy, physical therapy, respite providers, home health VNA, or whatever other services are needed or friends doing something.

Option one

I found that an actual calendar format was useful because I could see at a glance when I had appointments or when I needed coverage, and it was easier to make changes. The calendar format also permits VNA and other support staff to see the patient's schedule with a quick glance.

It enables you to check the calendar for other appointments to help you avoid multiple appointments at the same time. Sometimes, one specialist will want to see you after you've seen another. You simply pull out your manual and check the calendar for the appointment.

Another friend kept a Google calendar on her laptop.

Option two

Bob preferred a list so that each date is listed consecutively and appointments are written next to the appropriate date. The list format can allow space to write in the results of doctor's visit next to the appointment. However, I include any pertinent information in the question section of my manual.

Regardless of which format you choose, if you are unable to attend the doctor's visits with the patient, make sure that someone remembers to take notes of the session unless you are taping them. If you use option one, notes would go in the question and answer section. If you use option two, the notes would go next to the appointment.

Use whatever works for you.

The following situation that my friend Betsy was in shows how important a resource manual can be. She had to take her mother-in-law, Jean, who suffers from dementia, to a new neurologist. This was the first time Betsy had taken Jean to the doctor. Normally, Jean's daughter took her. When the neurologist wanted to know Jean's history, Betsy was unable to provide it. The neurologist had to contact Jean's primary care physician and present neurologist to gather the information. If Jean's daughter had a resource manual, Betsy could have brought it to the appointment, and saved everyone time.

It is important to have a record that is accessible to other family members in the event something happens to the primary caregiver or if caregiving is shared.

CALENDAR OF SOCIAL EVENTS FOR THOSE WITH IMPAIRED MEMORIES

Some patients, particularly those with impaired memories, may wish to keep their own social calendar of events. This calendar offers a place for them to keep track of visits from family members and friends, a kind of guest book in which visitors can log in or leave little notes or pictures. Together with the patient, you will want to decide whether this section belongs in your resource manual or on its own. Privacy, convenience, the size of your resource manual and the size of this section are important considerations in making this decision.

For children who cannot read a calendar with pictures may be helpful.

MEDICATION

List **current medication and allergies,** if any. Make columns to include the following information.

Include a detailed medication schedule including dosage and times to take it. You can use an F following each medication name to indicate that it should be taken with food or NF to indicate it should not be taken with food. Be sure to include both the generic and brand names. The name the doctor told you (often the brand name) and the name on the bottle, may be different, since the generic form is often provided.

It is important to realize that many medications come with unpleasant side effects which are not the same as an allergic reaction. Usually there is a sheet of paper with the medication which spells them out. For clarification, you can ask the pharmacist when you pick up the medication.

Many people find a pill box or med planner helpful and fill it weekly. They come in various sizes depending on needs. If your care recipient has more pills than the med planner will hold then you will need to devise your own system.

It is important that you know exactly what you are giving the patient. It is easy to become confused by the different names. That's one reason I found the log helpful.

Include the history of the use, purpose, reaction or response to the medication.

The following examples show some of the ways this chart can be used. Gerry's son, Henri, was diagnosed with schizophrenia. Gerry found it helpful to keep track of the different anti-psychotic medications and how they affected his son. In some cases the medication was not effective or the side effects were too distressing. The log helped when Henri was hospitalized and the new doctors wanted to try different medications because he was able to report accurately what had been tried and the results.

Samantha's doctor recommended using medication to help diminish her husband's combative behavior as a result of dementia. Samantha tracked her husband's behavior before and after medication and as the medication was increased. She was able to help the doctor find the optimum dosage for her husband based on her charts.

While her husband was having chemotherapy, Martha sometimes had to adjust her husband's medications. She kept a journal of how each day went and how much medication she gave him. She learned that when she gave him a whole pill, that he slept so much he wouldn't eat and he needed to eat to maintain his weight. She also tracked his blood pressure which the doctors wanted to know.

Helpful hint

The medication page is useful when a new medication is prescribed. It can help you to verify that there will be no interactions with current ones prescribed by a different specialty, and clarify that the present doctor is aware of all medications that your loved one is taking. Pharmacies also provide this information. For this reason it is helpful to use the same pharmacy for all prescriptions. Be sure to tell the pharmacist if the care receiver is taking any vitamin or herbal supplements or over-the-counter medications because they can also interact with prescribed medication.

QUESTIONS

I found this section was really important as it allowed me to compare notes and answers from different doctors about Bob's diagnosis, especially since doctors don't always agree.

It is a good place if you have questions about the medications, the side effects, the illness itself or what is to be expected from the illness and is another good reason to take your resource manual with you when you go to the doctor's.

Hint

As you think of questions between appointments, add them to this section. When you go to the doctor, your questions are there in front of you. Remember to write down the response and repeat it back in your own words. Do not be intimidated if you do not understand. Simply ask for clarification. Your doctor went to school to learn about medicine and the body and to learn the technical terms; it is not your responsibility to know this language automatically.

However, your loved one's diagnosis, response and changes in behavior are now your concern. You have a history and daily interaction with that person; the doctor does not. You are a conduit for information about him to the doctor. This is especially important if he has difficulty communicating or forgets to tell the doctors what changes have occurred between appointments.

When my mother was sick, she would often complain of symptoms at home, but when she was taken to the doctor, she would say she was fine. The family had to remind her to tell the doctor what she had been saying at home.

If someone else provides transportation to the doctor, be sure to advise that person or the patient, if able, to record the answers to the questions.

If you have difficulty listening and taking notes like I do, you can bring a mini-tape recorder and record your doctor's visits. This can provide a wonderful way of review-ing and clarifying what the doctor said.

HOSPITALIZATIONS

You will probably need a section on hospitalizations. In-clude reason for admission, dates, length of stay, proce-dure and results.

For example, if your loved one has cancer, you would record surgeries and other procedures. If the plan was to remove a tumor, document the location of the tumor, and whether or not the surgery was successful.

Or if an emergency hospitalization is required, note the reason. This may enable you to see a pattern and be pro-active in the future.

During the course of Bob's illness, he developed pneu-monia and pleurisy and needed to be taken to the hospital one night. I was able to provide the emergency room staff with information about his illness that they would not other-wise have known.

LABORATORY RESULTS - OPTIONAL

Depending on the diagnosis and the complications that arise, you may need a section with lab results. Many disor-ders rely on lab results to measure and/or diagnose.

For example, Al, who is HIV positive, keeps track of his lab results, particularly T-cells, to ascertain the progression of the illness and the resiliency of his immune system.

Sometimes the effectiveness of a medication is mea-sured by a lab value. For example, blood levels are mea-sured for some medications that are prescribed for people with mood disorders. This enables the doctor to see how a particular patient metabolizes a medication and to make sure that the patient has reached but not exceeded the therapeutic level. In some cases it can tell whether or not a patient is taking the prescribed medication.

If the doctors order a number of blood tests, you may want to ask what the purpose of the blood tests is and then obtain the result. Many doctors will provide their patient with a copy of the lab results if there is a need. (Incidentally you are entitled to copies of your medical records which clearly includes laboratory results.) Hole punch them and add them to the section. Since often there are labs that are not particularly pertinent, you can highlight the one(s) of concern. Or, you can create a graph to help you see a pattern (blanks can be downloaded from my website).

TRANSPORTATION – OPTIONAL

If you are relying on a number of different people to provide this service, then you may want a separate section.

An alternative is to incorporate it into the calendar section. The phone numbers of the persons providing the transportation could go on an individual sheet in the front after the doctors and other providers.

If the transportation is being coordinated through an organization or a church, then you would probably want to include the name of the person directing the service for you. Many organizations have volunteers who are willing to provide transportation and other services. For example, the American Cancer Society has volunteers who are willing to take people to their chemotherapy appointments. You would need to check with your local organization to determine if they provide that service and have anyone available when you need them.

I like to include the telephone number of the person providing the transportation, so that I don't have to research it if that person is late or I have a question.

If the doctor's office calls to change the appointment time, then I have the telephone number of the person immediately under the scheduled appointment. If there is sufficient time and transportation is coordinated through someone else or an agency such as the Council on Aging, then clearly that is whom you need to call.

In my case, I tried to attend all of Bob's doctor's appointments but we paid a neighbor to take Bob to his radiation appointments. I would not have been able to continue to work if I had been required at all of his radiation appointments. And, frankly, we needed my income to support us. After the acute phase of his illness, Bob began to drive himself until he had a non-convulsive seizure and was not permitted to drive for six months.

SPECIAL NEEDS OR HELPFUL HINTS FOR PROVIDERS - OPTIONAL

If your loved one has special needs or you have found certain techniques helpful, you will need a section for this. This is especially true if you have a number of support personnel coming in to be with your care recipient. They will need to know what works and what doesn't. If you have concerns about confidentiality and the provider is not a professional who would need to know, you may chose to have a separate notebook for this.

It may be as simple as your loved one is deaf in one ear so professionals coming need to know which side to be on to speak to your loved one and be heard. In Bob's case for example, he needed to have both hearing aides in to hear anyone. (I also completed a form for 911 which told responders that he would not be able to hear without his hearing aides. This was a form I got from the state. I did this so they would know to check for his hearing aides if I wasn't there to assist.)

If the providers coming into your home are new, you will certainly want to have a discussion with them about caring for your loved one and allow for an introductory period. If possible, and this may be a luxury, plan a meeting prior to the first paid visit.

If memory is an issue, this visit may not matter. But it will still provide you with an opportunity to see how the new care provider is going to interact with your loved one and vice versa.

INSURANCE

If your insurance requires co-pays and/or it is complicated and/or it is thru Medicare, then you may decide to have a separate binder for insurance. Many insurance companies including Medicare send out statements which are not bills but provide information about what procedure has been done, what the charge is, what the insurance has paid, and what your expected payment will be.

If you have more than one insurance, you will need to track the payments, who has been billed, what has been paid and by whom. The paperwork can sometimes be overwhelming. But if you organize it by insurance company and keep the statements together, it makes it easy to cross reference and create a paper trail. This can be one of the more challenging aspects of caregiving, particularly if paperwork is not your forte.

It will be easier if you keep up with it as it comes in or, if that is not possible, you need to set aside a particular time each week to review the forms, bills, etc. that have come in that week.

There are two ways you can file them in your binder. One is by buying a three-hole punch and punching the holes in each statement or bill as it comes in. The alternative way, which I think is really more cumbersome, is to buy the plastic holders and to put each new statement in its own plastic sleeve. There are also plastic folders which allow you to store loose material but this can be unwieldy. You may decide that a binder is not the solution and use file folders.

COPIES OF ADVANCE DIRECTIVES, LIVING WILLS, ETC.

If you are a caring for someone who is eighteen or older it is important for you to have copies of living wills or durable powers of attorney for health care or whatever particular health documents your state uses. It is important not only for the patient to have these forms completed but you should also complete these forms for yourself. These forms are discussed in greater detail in "Chapter 6, Finances and Legal Matters."

Depending on the family situation, you may want to talk with your family, friends, attorneys about making arrangements in case something should happen to you.

As you may have realized, your resource manual is a work in progress. It will continue to grow and at some point you will outgrow your original manual. By then you will probably have a good handle on caregiving, and you can decide whether or not you wish to continue. Part of this decision may be based on the number of support staff or helpers who come and care for your patient. If you do, you may need to keep the basics.

The following ideas, although not part of the resource manual, are important for caregivers to consider.

HELPFUL IN CASE OF EMERGENCY

It is vital to have the bare minimum of information about diagnosis, medications, doctors and living wills or durable power of attorney for health care in a plastic sheet easily accessible to the door in the event you need to call for emergency assistance; the first responders can be given the information as they arrive. During Hurricane Katrina many people's medical records were destroyed either in the hospitals that were flooded or in the doctors' offices. If you need to evacuate, it would be helpful for you to bring your resource manual with you – even though it will not contain a complete medical history – or if time is limited, the plastic sheet you keep by the door for emergency personnel. You may also want to store basic information on a flash drive to carry with you.

HELPING NON-VERBAL OR NEUROLOGICALLY IMPAIRED CHILDREN OR ADULTS

For children who can't yet read but can understand and point at pictures, you may wish to create, with your child, a book of pictures to point to ideas when she is not feeling well. This could include favorite foods, pictures representing pain or hurt with various parts of the body, requests they might have such as to watch a favorite movie or have a massage or to have the dog on the bed, if allowed. If your child has learned sign language – either her own or American Sign Language, your child signing could be some of the pictures. You could also include pictures (or images to remind her) of the visiting nurse or doctor if you want her to know when those visits will occur.

For older children and adults who may become impaired neurologically or have difficulty communicating, a similar book is suggested. It can be done when the diagnosis suggests that communication will become a problem so that the family can prepare together for the transition. Favorite foods, "scratch my back," "can we go for a walk," pictures about how the day is ("this day sucks!"), "Can you read to me," "My favorite show is on now," "I'm cold," "I'm hot." are all fodder for the book. Again a binder is suggested. It could be divided into sections for food, how your loved one is feeling, requests, information or any that you think appropriate.

As you can see there are lots of different kinds of information and ways of organizing it. Clearly, you must have what you need. The challenge when the caregiver is first starting out is to know what is and is not important. The Resource Manual gives you a place to start until it is clear.

CHAPTER 3

TAKING CARE OF OURSELVES

Importance of self-care

Caregiving can be an overwhelming job. When Bob was sick, I was so focused on him that I wasn't paying attention to my own needs. As soon as I thought he was better and I could relax a little, something else would happen. I realized that if I didn't take care of myself, I might get sick and not be able to care for him at all. I was not a limitless stream of energy and caring but rather a finite well. If I didn't take care of myself, I would run dry. I remembered caregivers from support groups who became sick. Their loved ones then had to be placed in nursing homes or respite beds until the caregiver was well again. I didn't want that happening to Bob.

I developed migraine headaches. I tried a number of different approaches ranging from support groups to acupuncture to massage to exercise to help relieve my stress and eliminate my migraines. It seemed I would be fine until Bob required another surgery for something. It didn't seem to matter to my head that a particular surgery was not cancer related or a fairly simple procedure. Although I had medication for the migraines, they seemed to hit as Bob was being wheeled into surgery and in some cases

I had the responsibility to drive him home post-surgery. The medication made me sleepy – not good for driving. Sleep was the best cure for the headaches but not possible when you're in a day surgery waiting room or at work.

Over time, I found increasing the supplements I took, walking our dog, getting a massage and taking hot baths worked best for me. I learned this through a process of elimination, trying what others suggested and what worked for them and seeing if it eased my stress.

It simply isn't easy to take care of ourselves and our loved ones. And what works for one person doesn't work for another. Often the care recipient's needs increase so gradually that by the time the caregiver realizes how overwhelmed she is, she has trouble figuring out how to care for herself. Caregivers worry that something will happen to the care recipient while they are caring for themselves. Often they feel they could not live with that guilt. It becomes a catch-22. A caregiver needs to maintain her own health in order to look after the care receiver yet the care receiver may need 24 hour supervision.

It is always a difficult decision and each one of us finds our own way to handle it. When possible, explore all of your options. The following are possible approaches to self-care. I recommend you scan the list to see what resonates with you and will fit into your schedule. For ongoing replenishment, use the ones that work best for you.

Support Groups

All groups offer a health benefit in providing a much-needed break for the caregiver.

Caregiver support groups provide an important way to gather information, get support, learn effective techniques for handling specific problems and share experiences.

- **Join** if one already exists.

  Often local hospitals, Councils on Aging, Area Agencies on Aging, adult day care programs, Visiting Nurse Associations and associations related to the particular diagnosis may offer such groups.

  Local papers may carry times and locations of meetings.

- **Start a group.**

  If a caregiver support group does not exist in your locale, you can start one, encourage the local hospital to, or find a caregiver chat room on line.

  If you decide to start a group, remember to share the responsibility for maintaining it with the other people who attend. Hospitals, churches and senior organizations will usually allow public meetings to be held for free.

- **Unusual diagnosis**

  If you are caring for someone with an unusual diagnosis, ask the doctor if he or she will post a notice (or permit you to) or pass out a flier or survey asking for contacts. You might even ask if there are a number of others with that diagnosis. Your doctor will not be able to provide you with a list of names due to confidentiality issues.

- **Finding a location**

  If the local hospital is not willing to start a group, they may be willing to provide a meeting room. Libraries and local community colleges often have meeting space available. Religious establishments and civic organizations may help with meeting rooms if they can.

If you are near an office of a non-profit group that is dedicated to that particular illness, they may offer support groups or be willing to host them. They may have a list of people who have enquired about support or be able to include your information in a newsletter.

- **Facilitator for the group**

    It is best to have someone other than yourself facilitate the group. If you cannot find someone to do that, then group members could take turns.

    Schools of social work, counseling or psychology might also be able to provide you with either professors, students or former students who might be willing to serve in some capacity and/or be able to direct you towards an agency that would. If your loved one is a senior citizen, councils on aging may offer ideas or locations.

Support groups for caregiver and patient

Depending on the diagnosis and the age of the loved one, you may choose to include him or her as part of the support group. I once facilitated a group of Parkinson's patients and their spouses. Not only did the patients learn practical tools to manage their disease, but their partners shared frustrations and concerns in providing care. This group was started by a patient, but led by a professional.

- **Chat rooms**

    Chat rooms or blogs may be helpful whether or not you attend a caregiver support group. The internet is a great resource, but remember to consider the source of any information. Of course, anyone can post any information they want on the internet whether or not it has been researched, is fraudulent or kooky so it is best to know the author or organization that you are using for information. You can find ideas, resources and approaches that you may be able to use. Perhaps an idea will surface that you can adapt to your circumstances.

- **Faith-based groups**

   Many people find support through their place of faith, not only by attending regularly-scheduled services but by groups that may be offered. A committed group that meets regularly can provide a respite from caregiving and/or work – if you also work outside the home.

   George was caring for his wife, Grace. They had been married 40 years and she now suffered from dementia. George found it challenging to remain upbeat but made it a point to attend a weekly group. "I enjoy going to the men's group at church. We start and end with a prayer. Sometimes it seems that's the only quiet time I have all week. I feel closer to God; I like the camaraderie with the guys and it provides a break from caring for Grace. My daughter comes and cares for Grace while I'm out."

- **Exercise Groups**

   In many areas, there are exercise, yoga, meditation, or tai chi groups that offer a regular opportunity to meet others and get an additional health benefit from these activities. Like support groups, most of these groups meet at a regularly scheduled time. They can offer a diversion without demanding too much involvement.

My husband and I did tai chi together through adult education at the local high school. The tai chi helped my stress and improved his balance, which had been affected by a brain tumor. See below for additional information about exercise.

- **Hobby groups**

If you presently enjoy a hobby, this may be a way to relax. In my area, for example, I know that there are spinners, weavers, and quilters who meet on a regular basis. Working with threads and yarn has been a timeless method of escape and repose. My friend, Samantha, finds crocheting very soothing. "There is something about the rhythmic, repetitive, meditative motion that calms my anxiety."

Stamp and coin collecting, toying with trains, gardening, playing a musical instrument or singing are just a few activities that people can do at home or in groups which provide solace while caregiving. Being able to enjoy your pastime at home and still care for your loved one is a bonus.

If you presently have a leisure pursuit or belong to a group that energizes you, this is probably not the time to give it up.

Prior to Bob's illness, I had provided respite care for my mother who had heart problems. In this case, the patient maintained her hobby. My mother was a bridge fiend and although she was not well enough to leave the house, her friends were kind enough to come and play with her, even after her skills deteriorated. It was fun for everyone and provided a break for her caregivers.

Exercise

Exercise relieves stress, lowers blood pressure, can increase the amount of energy you have and releases endorphins, our bodies' natural stress reliever. If you have an exercise program or a sport in which you participate already, you are ahead of the game. Maintaining that favorite pastime or program will enable you to be at your best when you need to be the caregiver. If not, you may want to consider joining a weekly group such as one of those mentioned above to get yourself started.

Even if your options for exercise are limited, small exercises which can be done in your chair will contribute to your well-being. In my area, public television offers exercises every morning at 6:30 am. Each day a different approach is provided and one of those days is for people who exercise in their chairs. There are also chair exercise videos available for purchase. The following web sites offer a selection of different videos and options: www.sitandbefit.org (based on the television series), www.armchairfitness.com , www.chairdancing. com, and www.peggycappy.com (offers yoga in a chair).

Jean likes to get up early in the morning and ride her stationery bicycle while she watches the morning news. Her husband is still sleeping so she is able to use that time without feeling guilty. And, in the winter, she gets refreshed seeing the sun come up outside her window.

I found that when I could go for a half hour walk when I was upset that after about ten minutes the reason would have disappeared or sometimes when I was searching for answers sometime along the walk I would figure out the solution. My challenge was that when Bob was well enough, he would want to come with me or we had to walk the dog. Although I enjoyed Bob's company as well as the dog's, the walk was not as therapeutic as when I went by myself. Bob could not walk as fast as I would like or for as long so often he would turn around and go home and I would spend the rest of the time wondering if I was going to find him collapsed on the road when I returned home.

Diet

Eating nutritional food is critical at this time. Caregiving is stressful and time consuming so there is always the temptation to eat junk food or fast food. Time to prepare healthy, nutritional meals seems non-existent. However, nourishing meals are important for both the loved one and caregiver.

Options to think about.

- Stores offer options now that can help. Bagged salads and pre-cut vegetables, for example, are a couple of easy ways to help you get your needed vegetables.
- More and more restaurants are offering meals to go. Some fast food chains are now providing healthier options.
- I have found it helpful to make enough for at least two meals and freeze the second meal. On a day when we know our schedule is tight, we thaw the second meal and heat it up.
- Or make something that can be used in a variety of ways throughout the week. For example, roast a chicken, use leftovers for chicken salad or chicken tetrazini.
- Crock pots can be a caregiver's best friend. I have even roasted chicken in my crock pot and it has been quite tender. Using crock pots in the summer helps to keep the house cooler and uses less electricity.

Respite Care

Most caregivers struggle with finding time to care for themselves. Caregiving requires juggling people, schedules and commitments when there are already forty balls in the air. However, some studies indicate that respite is not only helpful for the caregiver but also for the care recipient, even lowering the number of hospital admissions for the care recipient.

Caregivers may give up trying to find someone to provide respite or feel only they can provide the right care for their loved one. And, it is true that some of our loved ones get agitated or worse with new people. Conversely, others are actually better with non-family members. You cannot always gauge this by the first experience or by the first respite provider. Don't be afraid to persist if the first time does not go exactly as planned. It can be a bit like finding the right baby sitter for a cantankerous child.

Family members

Most caregivers look to other family members first. The reasons are obvious – relationship, familiarity and closeness. Family meetings can help clarify the patient's needs and provide an opportunity for family members to discuss solutions. However, families do not always live nearby, are not always available, may not wish to participate, or do not provide the best care. Family members may also be going through their own grieving process and express anger or denial about the situation towards siblings or parents. It is not unusual for this stressful time to elicit all of our past dysfunctional patterns. For this reason, I recommend that family members be gentle with each other.

Families who do not live nearby may be willing to travel and serve for a block of time. For example, my brother, Alan, and I both provided respite care for our mother, which enabled her caregivers (another brother, David, and his wife, Jill) to take an extended vacation. I also traveled from New Hampshire to New York to care for my mother every other weekend so David and Jill could get away.

Hospice

Hospice is a term used to describe care provided to patients at the end of their lives. It is intended to provide relief from pain and manage symptoms.

In order to receive hospice care, a physician must certify that the patient has a life expectancy of six months or less. Some insurances including Medicare Hospital Insurance (Part A) cover hospice. Most often this is provided at home although it can also be provided in nursing homes, hospice homes and hospitals. To clarify what is covered, it is best to call your insurance provider. Some respite care can be part of hospice coverage. If your loved one is already receiving hospice, it may be easier to talk directly with your provider. Sometimes if the care recipient is not in the active dying stage (See Chapter 1, page 10 for an explanation), there is a board and room charge.

Volunteers

Neighbors, friends, fellow parishioners from your place of faith should all be considered. Jean and her circle of friends wanted to be involved in the care of her best friend, Mary. George, Mary's husband, was initially resistant. He felt he should provide all of Mary's care. Jean arranged for Mary's friends to rotate a two-hour stint daily so that George could take a break. Each friend only had to be there once every two weeks. George found he liked the break and could check on his business. Mary took pleasure in seeing her friends and the friends found it a way to stay connected and be part of the process.

When fourteen year old Janelle was dying of cancer, her friends from school stayed with her while her Mom ran errands. Janelle had also met friends from cancer camp who lived close enough to drop by occasionally and boost her morale. Janelle liked seeing all of her friends and felt she didn't have to explain what she was going through to the other kids from camp. Her Mom was happy for the respite and to see her daughter enjoying some companionship during her last weeks.

Paid companions

Retirees and/or college/high school students may provide care although usually at a cost. It is important to be aware not only of your loved one's needs but also the capabilities of your respite providers.

Be sure to interview prospects if they are not known to you; also provide pertinent care information or special techniques that you have found work for you in caring for your loved one. Be clear about your loved one's needs, idiosyncrasies, and suggested coping strategies. These can be added to your resource manual (see Chapter 2).

Certified (or Licensed) Nursing Aides or Personal Care Attendants may be willing to work extra time. In some areas, there are agencies that will supply CNAs, PCAs and home health aides to provide respite. Some may be willing to assist with other duties such as shopping or light housework but clearly this falls under the category of homemaking and not companionship.

Some agencies provide companions who do not have any particular training, but who give wonderful respite care. These people are helpful when a loved one cannot be left alone and would also benefit from having someone other than the caregiver to talk to. Socialization can be important for all involved.

Fees for non-volunteers will need to be negotiated. Agencies may base fees on income and/or assets. Others may charge a set fee. Fees will also vary with the part of the country you live in.

It is important when you have someone providing assistance that you continue to monitor the situation. Unscrupulous individuals have sometimes taken advantage of some care recipients. In one instance, an elderly woman was beaten by one of the people an agency supplied. Family members were told the bruising was due to the blood thinner the patient was taking. Only after that patient's death did the truth come out. The family felt guilty that they had been so gullible. Others have lost money or jewelry. At the same time, there are many fine people who assist families in caring for their loved ones.

The Alzheimer's Association has a carefinder section on their website, www.alz.org/carefinder. Although it is clearly geared for those caring for someone with a memory disorder, it has some good tips and useful information.

Day programs

Day programs that encourage group activities may be available in your community. Many cities have adult day cares for seniors or disabled persons. These often provide nursing coverage, a meal, and supervision for a very nominal fee. Transportation is often available, although there may be a charge.

Company programs

One large company sponsored an adult day care that shared some activities and space with its child care program. Employees could take advantage of either. As our population ages, more companies may explore this option.

Mental health clinics.

If your loved one has a mental illness, exploring local services is important. Although mental health clinics have decreased services for eligible clients in recent years, you may be able to find a day program geared to mental health issues.

There are still a few "clubs" which mental health consumers run. They are intended primarily for socialization and do not offer structured activities. You may need to explore if transportation is available and if there is a cost. Check with your community mental health clinic to see what services are available. Often what services are provided depends on the severity and duration of the illness.

Diagnosis specific groups for the patient

Local hospitals or associations offer support groups for those with a specific diagnosis. These groups usually meet weekly for an hour or so and are only intended to provide support for the patient and/or family or caregiver. For example, a friend of mine attends a regular support group for survivors of lung cancer.

Nursing homes, assisted living facilities and respite care facilities

For a longer respite period, many long term care facilities will provide respite for a fee. Fees vary depending on the facility. Sally had been caring for her husband, Matthew, who had been diagnosed with Alzheimer's and suffered with paralysis on his right side. Sally's doctor recommended knee surgery. Sally was very reluctant to place Matthew in a nursing home while she had the surgery done. Sally continued to suffer with her knees until she slipped on the ice badly injuring one of them. She had to be hospitalized and Matthew was placed in a nursing home. During Sally's rehabilitation period, she was able to share a room with her husband although normally rehabilitation and longer term care were in different parts of the nursing home. She saw how much work it took for others to care for him. She realized she could no longer care for him at home when she noticed the number of people required to transfer Matthew from his bed to his chair.

Vacation Style Respite

Perhaps the best known of these is Paul Newman's Hole-in-the-Wall-Gang Camps (www.holeinthewallcamps.org)

where children who have cancer, HIV/AIDS, and other blood disorders can attend camp. Medical personnel are provided. This offers children who are too ill to go to a regular camp a place to go and meet similarly diagnosed children. Simultaneously, parents are provided with a much needed break while the children are at camp. Other weekend, summer and year-round camp programs are available. Since there are so many options from those for disabled vets to people with cerebral palsy, it is best to do your own search on Google, contact the local organization for the particular disorder, or speak to your librarian and ask him/her to research it for you.

Royal Caribbean Cruise Lines offers special packages for those who need specialized medical care such as dialysis. Contact the cruise line for more information.

State-Funded Respite Care

Some states offer family caregivers respite either through supportive funding of respite care or in some cases, through trained volunteers. For more information, see a state-by-state listing on the Family Caregiver Alliance Web site at www.caregiver.org.

The National Respite Coalition,

www.archrespite.org, offers a state-wide directory to assist caregivers to find respite. There are not always respite providers for all situations and when a provider is found, respite may not be available for the time needed.

Dial 2-1-1

United Way of America is hoping to make this number available nationwide to connect people with community services and volunteer agencies. At this time, only about 75 percent of Americans can use this number.

V.   Transportation.

Public transportation
Some local communities offer discounted transportation for seniors and/or disabled persons. In some states this is free.

Senior centers, Area Agencies on Aging, or Councils on Aging.
Many senior centers provide transportation for elders to medical appointments. Sometimes there is a fee associated with the transportation. In some states, part of the cost may be waived or paid by the state if you meet certain income requirements.

Local Chapters
Sometimes volunteers at local chapters of national organizations such as the American Cancer Society, National Hospice and Palliative Care Organization, Disabled American Veterans' Voluntary Service Program offer transportation. These opportunities are decreasing because of liability issues and available personnel.

Renal failure
Those with renal failure who are unable to drive themselves to dialysis may be eligible to have transportation reimbursed through insurance. You need to check with your insurance provider.

VI.   Alone time
Alone time can be as crucial as group support. This may be a time for prayer, reflection, meditation, exercise, yoga, or simply reading a book or magazine.

I find sitting in a warm bath, with the light from a couple of candles, a favorite book or a glass of wine incredibly soothing. Sometimes, I don't read, I just enjoy the atmosphere.

Ginny loves to run and finds a way to squeeze it into most days. Sometimes, it's first thing in the morning if she wakes up before the rest of the household; other times it's while her husband is taking a nap.

When Molly's best friend was dying of cancer, the only time she found solace was weeding the garden. There was something about the meticulousness of differentiating weeds from vegetables. It was something she had control over.

Tapes and CDs

Guided imagery tapes and CD's are available that are specifically intended to help relieve stress. Guided imagery is imagining what someone is telling you. You can find some relaxing CDs at the local store under such categories as nature, new age or meditation. HealthJourneys, an organization that specializes in guided imagery, is accessible on the web and offers a variety of tapes and CDs. It can be found at www.healthjourneys.com. They have ones to relieve stress and many that are disease specific. The guided imagery which is found at the end of the book and was created for caregivers may be downloaded free from my website, www.joanperry.net using the user name, caregiver, and the password, imagery. (These are case sensitive so use lower case letters.) Look for the button on the home page and click on that.

Stress management

Many options exist to help you deal with stress and buoy up your immune system. If you are unsure about exploring these options, you can discuss them with your doctor or someone who has used them.

- **Massage and Energy Work** are two of my favorites. You need to find someone with whom you feel comfortable and whose style matches your needs. There are many different kinds of body work and massage therapists often combine an eclectic approach in working with a client. The most common forms of massage are Swedish, deep tissue, hot stone, Shiatsu and Thai. Because of the variety of practitioners and the services they offer, they are more than willing to explain how they work. And like choosing any professional, you need to find one that makes you comfortable.

For those who are not at ease being naked under a sheet other options may include energy work such as Reiki, Integrated Energy Therapy® and craniosacral therapy. These are alternative practices based on the premise of a human energy field or life force around the body. They use a form of laying on of hands to correct imbalances which impact our life. Reiki and IET® are performed directly on the clothed person on an energy table. However, they can be done sitting up or at a distance.

Massage therapists as well as an extensive listing of types of massage and energy work can be found at www.massagetherapy. com or look in your local paper or telephone book. IET® practitioners can be found at www. learnIET.com.

- **Aromatherapy**

  Aromatic essences from plants are used to balance, harmonize and promote the health of body, mind and spirit. The essential oils may be used in the bath, massaged into the skin, inhaled directly, or used to scent the entire room. Aromatherapy is used for pain relief, stress and fatigue reduction and the alleviation of anxiety. The smell bypasses the conscious mind and thus directly stimulates the brain and the nervous system. Because of my allergies I avoided aromatherapy for a long time, then I learned that most do not trigger my allergies. The scents are too subtle.

Some cultures use aromatherapy in the work place to increase production and to provide a stress-free environment.

- **Acupuncture**

This ancient Chinese approach to prevention of illness by balancing the chi (or life force) surrounding the body has become more popular in the west recently. It is used to reduce stress, alleviate pain, and increase immunity. Sterilized needles are placed on meridians of the body based on the specific symptoms or area of concern. Although I am needle-phobic, I've found the treatments to be relaxing. Even though they are inserted into the skin, they do not hurt. They are not being used to inject anything and appear to be just barely under the skin. This may be an option that both caregiver and patient can use.

Charles started acupuncture to relieve his stress but now maintains that it has eliminated or at least controlled his allergies. He goes regularly and gets very upset when his acupuncturist has the nerve to go on vacation.

To learn more about acupuncture, visit www.nccarn.nih.gov.

- **Simultaneous treatment**

Many options can work both for the caregiver and the patient. Both can go to the same clinic and while one gets acupuncture, the other gets a massage. It can afford a guilt free breathing space for the caregiver while providing an opportunity for relaxation and enjoyment for the patient. Mary, who cared for her sister, Jen, took her when she went for a massage. Jen's appointment for Reiki was scheduled to end fifteen minutes after Mary's. This enabled Mary to relax and get the full benefit of her massage. Jen was delighted to be included in the excursion and also loved the time with someone other than family.

- **Natural/herbal remedies and supplements**

    There are many natural remedies and herbs that some have found helpful. Bach flower remedies are one such possibility. (The Bach flower remedies are dilutions of flower materials in a mixture of water and brandy. Because they are extremely dilute they do not have the taste or scent of the flowers used. They are based on similar ideas to homeopathic medicine except that all are derived from non-toxic substances and use the energies of the plants to alleviate problems.)

    To learn what would best suit your purpose, ask a professional in the field. Because many natural remedies can interfere with prescription medication, make sure you check with your doctor to make sure what you want to take will not interfere with any medication you may be prescribed.

    This is not the time to stop your vitamins. B vitamins, for example, help the body to deal with stress.

- **EFT (Emotional Freedom Techniques)**

    This is a technique that uses tapping on the meridians used in acupuncture. Gary Craig, the founder of EFT, wanted as many people as possible to be able to avail themselves of this technique but he has retired. You can still download DVD's or free information from the website www.eftuniverse.com. My own bias is if you want to use it that initially you need to find a practitioner who has been using it for a while when you first start. If afterward, you wish to continue on your own, that is fine. Initially, I believe it is helpful to have someone who can guide you through the process. Some will do EFT with you over the telephone. That being said it is a very powerful technique and has had amazing results from helping people with MS (multiple sclerosis) to migraine headaches to trauma issues to depression.

VI.   Friends and other social supports

Friends help us get through times like this. My friends and the people I worked with are largely responsible for holding me together during Bob's illness. I am so grateful for their presence and willingness to listen, even when all they heard was the silence on the phone because I was too upset to talk but needed to know they were there.

VII.   Meditation, Prayer, and Faith

There is evidence that meditation, prayer and faith all provide assistance to patient and caregiver. Continuing a religious or spiritual practice is another way of getting support and relieving stress. If you attend a place of worship, it is a great place to find solace and caring, concerned people.

My faith and meditation practice buoyed me up at my lowest times. Prayer and meditation can be done almost anywhere and for almost any length of time. If you use public transportation, you can do it while you ride to your destination. These can calm you down and keep you centered.

And don't forget to breathe! Sometimes just taking a deep breath can allow a short break and enable us to be reenergized. Some forms of meditation and guided imagery use a focus on the breath.

When driving yourself, it may not be a good idea to meditate because meditation often has a different focus and you can lose your concentration on the road.

VIII. Pets

For those of us who are animal lovers, pets can offer stress relief, joy and humor to our lives. Taking a walk with the family dog can provide some exercise as well as some needed respite. For some, stroking a cat or petting the dog is soothing and relaxing and can lower your blood pressure. And, a cat purring in your lap is incredible!

For others of us taking care of a pet may just be one more thing to do. This could be the time to take your neighbors up on their offers of help and ask them to walk the dog. However, if you don't have a pet presently, now is probably not a good time to introduce another dependent into your family life. If you're like many caregivers, you will also end up taking care of the family pet. An aquarium full of green scum and gasping fish will not lower your blood pressure!

IX. Sense of humor

Finally, it is vital to maintain your sense of humor and find the funny side in even the most stressful situations. Cry when you need to and laugh when you can. Studies have shown that a sense of humor helps to relieve stress, provides a heart workout, increases your immune system and relaxes your muscles. Researchers at Loma Linda University of Medicine have found that it helps protect the upper respiratory tract.

Laughter will help everyone. It improves relationships when you can find common ground for laughter and joy. You will feel better if you are happier and can be a better caregiver. Laughter can accomplish that.

Bob's sense of humor helped us through many times. My brother, David, and his wife came to visit us the Christmas shortly after Bob's surgery. The friend we were staying with had an enormous collection of mugs. Bob had selected a mug without paying attention to its inscription. David began reading, "Pardon me, but you've obviously mistaken me for someone who gives a shit." Bob looked crushed and turned to look at David. I said, "Bob, it's on the mug." "Oh," he said and then he began to laugh. As did we all.

It may be helpful to look for humor not only in your daily interactions and occurrences but also to seek sources such as movies or television that you both might enjoy together. Reading funny stories is another way to share laughter. Your local librarian can be a wonderful resource to help you find books, magazines, movies, or tapes that can provide humor. Perhaps reading the comics in the newspaper is more your style.

If you work outside the home, sharing funny experiences from work can help the family member stay in touch with that part of your life. Day care may be another source of humorous stories.

Laughter and a good sense of humor can also help deflect difficult questions until you have time to think about how you want to answer.

Regardless of your preference and style, taking care of yourself is important. Yet finding time for self-care is often challenging. If all else fails, you can help yourself by remembering to <u>breathe</u>. Since you're breathing anyway, a few moments of deeper, conscious breathing can work wonders.

CHAPTER 4

KNOWLEDGE IS POWER!

When Bob was diagnosed with a brain tumor (a skin cancer that had spread to his brain), I was lucky because I was working in a hospital and gleaned all the information I could from the doctors, the nurses and the library. I wanted to know what other treatments might be available and what options he would have if it spread elsewhere. The information was not good. Metastatic melanoma did not have a good prognosis. I have always preferred to know what I am facing. It helps me to cope. That is one reason support groups related to a particular diagnosis are so helpful for us.

Being a caregiver is a difficult passage in our lives. We end up learning about things most of us have never even thought about. It is necessary to learn about the medical condition, the financial implications, the legal facts and the best way to care for our loved ones and ourselves during a very trying time.

First, learn everything you can about the medical challenge you are facing. Often, there are other manifestations of an illness or other diagnoses that occur at the same time, or medically speaking, a co-morbid diagnosis. Next, discover if the illness is systemic (impacts the entire body) like multiple sclerosis or is localized (just in one part of the body) like thyroid cancer. Unfortunately, a heart problem may only be in the heart but it has an impact on the rest of the body and consequently, the person for whom you are caring. However, if the care recipient has two diagnoses either of which would be a problem, then it is even more important for you to do your homework.

So, where can you get information?

Doctors and hospitals

Your first source is your doctor who provided the diagnosis or the specialist to whom you have been referred. Pick his/her brain. A hospital library can provide a wealth of information. If it is too technical, skip it. You have enough to deal with; don't try to go to medical school too! Gather what you can that's useful and go on to other sources.

When you're visiting your loved one in the hospital, particularly if it is in a specialized area of a hospital, don't be intimidated to ask questions of the staff. Often on dedicated units, the nurses who are there have become experts in that particular area over time and may be able to address your questions in a language you understand. You can ask for a family meeting with the doctor, nurse or social worker to discuss concerns that you may have. However, remember to be prompt and have your questions prepared. Like you, they have limited time and will be more responsive if you are ready. You may want to ask if there is a specific association that can provide additional information or resources.

Organizations focusing on the disease/disability

Check out the organizations that are affiliated with the illness; they can provide you with helpful information. If it is fairly common, there will usually be an 800 number in the phone book. If you don't find the organization listed in the telephone book, ask your local librarian to locate the appropriate name and way to contact them. You can always check the internet. Most public libraries now have access time available. Usually you have to be a cardholder in that library and sign up in advance for the time slot you want. If you know that it is a rare disease, you can check for information through the National Organization for Rare Disorders, www.rarediseases.org or by toll free at 1-800-999-NORD.

When checking out web sites, be very specific about the diagnosis. For example, you may start with cancer but it will be more effective and informative if you look up the exact name of the diagnosis. The web site you select may require an exact spelling. I looked up basal cell carcinoma in the American Cancer Society's web site, www.cancer.org and got information. When I misspelled it using basel cell carcinoma, nothing came up. Even though The American Cancer Society has its own web site, many of the particular kinds of cancer have their own organizations and information. Of course, you may have to use your favorite search engine to get to the organization that will be helpful. If you're not computer savvy, ask assistance from a friend who is or if using a library's computer, ask one of the librarians. You may be able to find a chat group about the illness. Remember, anyone can go on a chat line so information can be invalid or unreliable. Information on Wikepedia can be changed or updated by anyone so may not be accurate.

Support Group

If you belong to a support group that is focused on a particular issue, ask other members about their experiences. The caveat here is that what happened to them or to someone on a chat site may not be universal or related to the specific disease you are interested in.

Medication

It is important for the caregiver to have an understanding of medication, its side effects, and possible reactions. Your pharmacist and doctor are your best resources. Information is usually provided with all prescription medication. A number of resources are available on the internet. Drug companies have web sites where you can look for information about their products. The National Library of Medicine in conjunction with the National Institute for Health offer the following website for medication information http://www.nlm.nih.gov/medlineplus/druginformation.html. Information may be accessed by using either the generic or the brand name of the drug.

Assistive technology

There is a vast array of assistive devices to help care recipients and caregivers, from clothing that uses Velcro for people who cannot use buttons or zippers to utensils to help people pull up their socks in the morning. When the care recipient is hospitalized, the physical therapist, occupational therapist, social worker or case manager may suggest helpful equipment or a different approach to provide care. If they don't, feel free to ask. For example, if you are being asked to monitor your child's diabetes, make sure you are trained. The nurse caring for your child can provide you with diabetes training. Additionally, you can request that a visiting nurse come to the home to verify that you are doing it correctly.

Another source of information can be a medical supply company. They sell and lease durable medical equipment (DME) which is equipment that is intended for repeated, medical use. Oxygen tanks, wheelchairs, prosthetics, hospital beds are a few examples. If the care recipient has insurance, check to see if insurance will cover part of the cost. Medicare sometimes pays 80% of the cost for DME so be sure to ask your doctor or the case manager/social worker at the hospital if what is ordered is covered. You can also check Medicare's web site or call 1-800-MEDICARE. Some medical supply companies offer more than DME and may be a resource for other helpful needs. Some provide clothing for people who may have difficulty getting dressed and need clothing that uses Velcro.

Some charities or Councils on Aging sometimes have durable medical equipment that you may borrow. You just need to return it when you no longer need it.

There may additional supplies that you will need that are not considered DME. For example, bandages and rubber gloves are not considered durable medical equipment. Remember to check with your insurance company to verify what they will cover.

Home modifications

There are many home modifications that may be necessary. Beds or doors equipped with alarms, ramps, wheelchair access to bathrooms/bedrooms/house are a few. If you need to modify your home and cannot afford it, check with the social worker at the hospital to see if there is an organization that provides assistance or will install it for you. If the social worker does not know, don't assume that there isn't one. Check with local non-profits to see if they can help. If you are a member of a congregation, some places of faith may be willing to assist. Call organizations that work with people with disabilities to see if your state provides this type of assistance to those with disabilities. Sometimes the process of finding help seems to be more frustrating than the assistance is worth; it can be discouraging and time consuming but necessary. This is especially difficult if you are also working outside the home. (Depending on your job, this may be a good time to consider telecommuting or using family leave time, if you are eligible. Bear in mind that if your loved one has a progressive disease you may need to keep working until it is absolutely necessary to use leave time.)

Caregiver training

When I decided to be a social worker, it was in part to avoid nursing. I am needle phobic and don't like seeing blood. Yet during Bob's illness, I have found myself learning and performing many actions that I certainly thought of as nursing care. And depending on the diagnosis and prognosis, you may find that you need training to lift or bathe a person. You do not want to injure your back and be unable to provide care because you tried to move someone improperly. You may want to consider some kind of mechanical patient lifter. You may have to learn techniques for managing behavioral challenges. Other areas that can come up are:

Monitoring diabetes

Responding to a seizure

Assisting someone to transfer from bed to commode or chair

Turning a patient to avoid bed sores

Monitoring skin breakdown

Changing bandages

Giving bedpans or urinals or emptying catheter bags

Cleaning someone who is incontinent of feces and/or urine

Keeping an eye on symptoms

Some caregivers provide physical therapy when the insurance says it will no longer pay. Before you do any of these, ask for training from the staff that routinely provides the service.

Rehabilitation and nursing homes

Some rehabilitation is done in hospitals. If more extensive therapy is required, patients may be transferred to a skilled unit of a nursing home or a rehabilitation center to undergo rehabilitation therapy. In some states, nursing homes do not provide rehabilitation; only designated facilities do.

Sometimes our loved one wants to come home before he is able and that puts a lot of pressure on us. When one of my uncles broke his hip and was in the rehabilitation part of a nursing home (this is usually referred to as skilled nursing care), I went to visit him. He could not yet accomplish many of the activities that physical therapy felt he should be able to do before he was discharged. All he saw was that he was in a nursing home and wanted to get out. And like many, he felt that people were sent to nursing homes to die. I told him that even though I understood his adamant desire to go home that the staff where he was receiving rehabilitation services was trained and skilled in caring for him and that he should wait until he was better, that his daughter, my cousin, would certainly do the best she could but that she didn't have the training to care for him. He decided to leave shortly thereafter against the advise of the staff. Later, when I visited him at my cousin's home, my uncle surprisingly confessed to me that indeed he had left the nursing home too soon.

By the same token, many caregivers wait too long to consider placement for their loved ones. If the care you are giving seems a bit much, it may be time to consider a more appropriate placement. Many caregivers expect that the stress will decrease when their loved one is placed. This may not always be the case. Sometimes a loved one deteriorates on placement and we feel guilty that we did that to them. Sometimes visiting them is challenging and leaving them at the end of a visit can be especially hard. When I visited my aunt in a nursing home, she would cry for joy when I came, weep while I was there and cry out of despair when I began to leave. These types of visits tear at our heartstrings and make us question whether we should visit at all. Each of us must decide that for ourselves and because circumstances differ widely there is no one answer.

At one time during my own caregiving stint, Bob was hospitalized with a very serious infection with temperatures as high as 103.4F. As a result he was very weak, required a walker and needed rehab. He always talked about wanting to come home and I wanted him home. I knew that for much of that time he was not ready or able to be at home. I found it necessary to form an alliance with one of the nurses to insure that he received the care that I wanted and for the most part, he was well cared for at the nursing home.

Like most employees, the people who are employed at nursing homes have a wide range of skills and professionalism. They can be awful or incredible and everything in between. Most of them work very hard for very little money. I found it helpful to be a presence there and to know the staff. In one instance, I questioned why he was not being given a particular medication which he needed. The nurse checked and got it ordered. It could easily have happened the other way. He may have been scheduled to take a medication which he shouldn't. Nurses are human too so be sure to speak up if you have questions. You don't have to be aggressive; simply ask a polite question. If you are not satisfied, ask for clarification. Have a dialogue not a fight. The fact that Bob, even when sick, was a delightful human being also impacted people's desire to care for him. In that regard, we were both fortunate.

I have learned so much that I never thought I would need to know and I'm sure all caregivers do. You may have started caregiving with little knowledge, however, by the time you have completed your journey you will have learned a lot! Some of the information you may actively seek to know but some of it you learn as you go along almost like osmosis. I try to think of this element of caregiving as an adventure in which I have an opportunity to learn and grow and this aspect, like the passage through our emotional challenges, is another part of the process.

CHAPTER 5

LET ME KNOW IF THERE IS ANYTHING I CAN DO FOR YOU.

I have always been blessed with thoughtful, generous and helpful friends. However, like many caregivers, I was reluctant to accept help. I felt I should be able to do it on my own and I didn't want to impose. Caregiving unfortunately can become an isolating and overwhelming task. I learned that accepting a gift can be harder than giving. Accepting a friend's contribution and allowing people who love us to participate in our lives is a gift for all concerned. For some, this may be the only way they can participate in your life so it is okay to allow them the gift of showing they care. Permitting others to assist helped me to take care of myself.

I found I could differentiate between those who sincerely wanted to be involved and those who just said it because they weren't sure what else to say. There are some who truly desire to help and don't know how or fear getting sucked into a situation that could be overwhelming. So they give us a hug and say, "let me know if there is anything I can do for you" as they make their way out the door.

Sometimes we cannot even voice or think what those needs might be. Our closest friends may be at a loss to figure out what to do. We don't know how to ask for help even when someone says, "What can I do for you?" That was the situation I found myself in when I was caught in the maelstrom of caring for Bob. For those who were concerned about us, I learned to be gracious and accept their gift of giving so that they could participate in caring for someone they also loved. When someone said, "let me know if there is anything I can do for you" I gratefully accepted. If they weren't sure what to do, I might say, "Could you please pick me up a couple of things at the store when you go?" or "Could you please drop off the dry cleaning when you're in town?" or whatever else I might need if I knew they were going to be in the area to do the errand.

The following is a list of services, some small, some large, that friends and relatives might do for us. Tasks can be done once or more frequently. Breaking up tasks sets definable limits, which can serve to reassure those who might fear becoming subsumed or whose time is limited but still want to help. Some people want to assist and lack time but are willing to use their financial resources. It is okay to accept those gifts as we would any other. However, if you are hesitant to suggest those kinds of contributions, you can make up a list or show them this list in the book, perhaps with your favorite ideas highlighted. I have not included items that might be a friend's special gift such as playing the harp, singing songs, reviewing/explaining the bills, or fixing the computer. Many churches offer communion or visitors to those who are home-bound.

ERRANDS

Grocery shopping or going to the farmer's market.
Pick up/drop off dry cleaning.
Take loved one to appointments, for rides, out for a treat, hairdresser/barber, etc.

Pick up/drop off library books/videos/DVDs.
Chauffeur children or other family members.
Pick up/drop off mail.
Do dump/recycling center runs.
Drop off/pick up car at repair shop.

OTHER TASKS

Do the laundry.
Make phone calls – disseminate information.
Update www.carepages.com or www.caringbridge.org – these are websites where caregivers can post information about a loved one rather than needing to call everyone. (And people who read the updates can also send messages. The caregivers can also find reading those messages uplifting.)
Write letters.
Read aloud – letters, books, etc..
Cook a meal (alone or with a group) or favorite dish. (Ask about dietary restrictions or problems eating.)
Create "frozen dinners" of favorite meals.
Order and deliver take-out from a restaurant.
Water garden/plants – (or give them foster care.)
Polish shoes.
Iron.
Arrange to clean the house (alone or with a group), or pay for such a service as a gift.
Clean the bathroom.
Mow lawn.
Trim hedges.
Weed/plant garden.
Till garden.
Shovel snow.
Take out garbage.
Clean car.
Sweep/clean garage/basement.
Do dishes.

PETS

Walk the animal.

Feed the animal(s).

Groom or comb the pet.

Cut toenails (if this is my cat or dog you are very brave).

Clean stall or cage or kitty litter.

Pick up poop from back yard.

Take animal to vet.

Provide respite or foster care.

If hospital/hospice/nursing home permits, bring pet for visit.

RESPITE (is an opportunity for the caregiver to come up for air)

Stay with care recipient while caregiver runs errands/goes to a spa/hairdresser/etc.

Offer (or arrange for) care so caregiver can go away for a day/night/weekend.

Pay for a massage for caregiver or care receiver.

Watch the house/pets/plants while patient and caregiver go away for a weekend/night/day/or longer.

Invite the children to stay at your house for day/night/weekend.

Host extended family.

Provide transportation to/from an adult day care.

Have patient stay with you until caregiver gets home from work.

GIFTS

A book (Generally something that doesn't require long concentration.)

Magazines/ crossword or other puzzle books.

Yarn for knitting/crocheting if that is an interest.

Relaxation tapes.

Gift certificate to a restaurant.

Game for the computer.

CDs or videos/DVDs.
Telephone card.
Fill up the car with gas.
Just listen.
Games. (Maybe a new favorite of yours to play with them.)
Share jokes or favorite humorous stories.

LONG DISTANCE HELPERS

Even those who do not live nearby can assist. Here are some ideas for them.

Research the illness/respite availability/facilities/benefits.
Write thank you notes.
Advocate with the insurance provider or clarify bills.
Check in on a regular basis.
Talk to caregiver/care recipient on the phone as a break.
Share jokes or other humorous stories.
Make phone calls – disseminate information and up-dates.
Call a restaurant that they both love and have a meal delivered.

CHAPTER 6

FINANCES & LEGAL MATTERS

When Bob was diagnosed with a brain tumor, the last thing I thought about was legal or financial issues. I wanted the doctors to do all that was possible to save him. However, shortly after we learned the dreadful news, we needed to make decisions about concerns we had never considered. Fortunately, we had our wills made out and Bob immediately completed and signed a living will and a durable power of attorney for health care, the advance directives required for our state in the event he was unable to make his own decisions.

Advance directives provide instructions regarding your future medical care.

A Florida case in 2005 raised the awareness of the need to make our desires known in writing. Terri Schiavo was twenty-six when she collapsed from heart failure in her home. The subsequent lack of oxygen led to severe brain damage. Eventually, her husband and parents became involved in a legal battle to determine what should happen to her. Her husband stated that she would not want to be kept alive by means of a feeding tube and advocated for the removal of the feeding tube, thus allowing her to die. Her parents felt that she was still alive and the feeding tube should remain. The case attracted significant media, political and legal attention including the Supreme Court and the State of Florida legislature before her husband was given authority to have the feeding tube removed. She died when she was forty-one.

This case has helped make us aware of how important it is for all of us over the age of eighteen to consider what we would want done in similar circumstances. Taking care of these documents can avoid battles later and is another way to care for ourselves as well. There are many variables we need to mull over. State laws vary, thus options can be different. You will need to confirm what your current state laws are. The following alternatives are not legal advice. For that, you need to consult an attorney in the state in which you reside.

ADVANCE CARE PLANNING

It is wise for each of us to plan what type of medical care we would want if we were unable to communicate our wishes to our family and healthcare providers. We need to think seriously about what we want. That sounds easy and it may be. You may feel that regardless of what happens you want the medical profession to do what it can to keep you or your loved one alive. That means that you could be kept on a ventilator (something which breathes for you), you could receive both nutrition and hydration (liquid) through a tube, etc. and be unconscious.

Before making a decision, it is helpful to sit down with your family and discuss the situation. Caregiver and care recipient should both have a health care plan and a legal plan. Remember to make provisions in case something happens to the caregiver. It is not unusual for caregivers to require hospitalization, leaving the care recipient home alone. (See Chapter 3, "Keeping Your Well Primed" for tips on dealing with stress. Being proactive about your health can help prevent the need for hospitalization.)

Some people are hesitant to discuss these issues for fear that it will somehow jinx the person or bring about death. Some avoid it because it means facing our own mortality. Family conversations about this can help relieve stress and family division if a family member does have a life-threatening illness.

There are a number of key terms used when discussing end-of-life issues. Artificial feeding and artificial hydration are used to describe receiving the necessary nutrients and liquids to sustain life, which are administered through some kind of tube into the body. Neither of these refers to the natural process of eating and drinking. There is little, if any, discomfort associated with artificial feeding or artificial hydration. It is natural for us to want to feed our families, so it is important to have a discussion about whether or not that is your wish. Some strongly advocate for continued feeding and hydration. Another viewpoint supported by The American Academy of Hospice and Palliative Medicine states that "when a person is approaching death, the provision of artificial hydration and nutrition is potentially harmful and may provide little or no benefit to the patient and at times may make the period of dying more uncomfortable for both patient and family." (http://www.aahpm.org/positions/nutrition.html, June, 2006)

Palliative care is care focused on relieving pain. Although it is provided for dying patients, it is given to any patient who requires it. It is intended to relieve pain while trying to maintain quality of life. It is a patient- and family-centered approach that uses an interdisciplinary team to deal with the comprehensive needs of both patient and family.

Life-sustaining treatment is defined as procedures without which a person would die. This can include cardiopulmonary resuscitation (CPR), mechanical respiration (a machine breathes for you), or kidney dialysis (a machine cleans your blood of toxins). It can also include the use of other external mechanical and technological devices, drugs to maintain blood pressure, blood transfusions and antibiotics. CPR involves the use of external chest compressions to stimulate the heart to start beating. Sometimes a defibrillator is used. (You may recognize that from the television shows where they put paddles on someone's chest and then ask everyone to stand clear.)

Once you have the family discussion and have agreed on a plan, it is necessary to complete the forms and have them witnessed and, in most states, notarized. In some states attorneys must complete the forms. They become your advance care directives. These documents indicate how you want to be treated medically, if you are unable to communicate those wishes. The advances in medical technology and the litigiousness of our society have made this more of an issue in recent years.

When your decision has been made, you then need to communicate your desires to your primary care physician, i.e. your main doctor, in the event a critical decision is necessary. You should provide a photocopy of the completed paperwork. It is important to tell all of your doctors and give each of them a copy of your advance directives.

ADVANCE CARE DIRECTIVES

There are two documents that tend to be used; one is a living will and the other is a durable power of attorney for health care. However, in some states, other documents can be used. For this reason, if you travel frequently between two states, you may want to verify that the document you create is valid in both states. Usually a healthcare provider will honor the document to the extent permitted by local law. www.putitinwriting.org is a web site provided by the American Hospital Association and provides links to advance directives for every state as well as a glossary of terms. It also has a wallet identification that you can print out, complete and carry indicating that you have discussed advanced directives with your family and providing names and addresses.

A **living will** – which can also be called a declaration, instruction directive or wishes for terminal illness - conveys your desires about life-sustaining treatments, if you are unable to speak for yourself and you are permanently unconscious or terminally ill. Most states require that two doctors record a terminal diagnosis in your medical records before the living will can be activated. The standard forms provide a starting point, but you may add additional details if you like. Many hospitals offer patients an opportunity to create one prior to surgery or other procedures.

A **durable power of attorney for health care** – which can also be called healthcare agent, proxy, representative or surrogate – is a document in which you name the person you trust to make healthcare decisions for you if you are unable either to communicate or make those decisions. Unlike the living will, most states will allow the healthcare proxy to act for you any time that you are unable to communicate for yourself. Unlike the living will, you don't have to be diagnosed with a terminal condition.

The **do not resuscitate** (DNR) order indicates that if you stop breathing or your heart stops, no attempt will be made to restart your breathing or your heart. Normally, resuscitation involves chest compression, defibrillator shock, insertion of a breathing tube and/or medication. Whereas defibrillators were originally only available in a hospital setting, they are becoming more common and are often available in public places and often carried in ambulances and police cars.

Many people believe that if they have indicated in their advance directive that they do not wish to be resuscitated if their heart stops or they stop breathing, then the ambulance or hospital will automatically follow those wishes.

There are two parts to this. One is that those desires must be communicated to the personnel who come in the ambulance and to the doctor in the hospital. During emergencies, it is natural for us to call 911 and thus emergency personnel will come to our door. Some EMTs (emergency medical technicians who are a part of ambulance staff) may question why you called them if you do not want the patient resuscitated. You may be unclear how ill your loved one is. Some institutions such as visiting nurse associations have forms (called portable DNR's) available which can be signed by your doctor indicating that you or the care recipient is a DNR and which may be kept in your home.

In some locations, it may be necessary to call police who call a medical examiner to pronounce someone dead. If the care recipient is transported to the hospital, the doctor or nurse practitioner must write DNR as an order in your chart each time a patient is admitted. If you are involved with hospice, it would be wise to check with the coordinating agency so that you know the proper procedure in advance.

When you have surgery, the permission you grant often suspends these documents until after the surgery. This allows the surgical staff to respond appropriately during surgery.

FINANCIAL PLANNING

What kind of financial planning you do depends on your means and to some extent on your insurance and age. I have included a broad range of possibilities. Not all will apply to each situation. If you have not been involved in the financial planning aspect of the relationship or find it stressful, consider finding a trusted friend to help or go with you. It is important when a person is diagnosed with a chronic or potentially life-threatening illness, that the spouse learn as much as possible about the finances, particularly if the caregiver has not been involved in the finances before. Caregivers caring for someone other than a spouse may or may not be involved in the finances. For example, a caregiver may be caring for a parent and another family member is handling the finances. Clearly, communication between the parties will be key. Caregivers need to know what insurance and financial limitations there may be.

Disability Benefits

Social Security pays two kinds of disability benefits. One is for those people with a medical condition that is expected to last for at least one year or result in death and who have worked the required amount of time when they become disabled. This is called Social Security Disability Insurance. To receive this benefit you must meet their criteria by having earned sufficient credits, working recently enough and having a medically disabling condition. Since the way that Social Security calculates all of this is very complicated, it is best to talk with them directly or go to their web site.

For clarification, visit their web site, www.ssa.gov or call the toll free number for Social Security is 1-800-772-1213. For deaf or hard-of-hearing, the TTY number is 1-800-325-0778.

The second is Supplemental Security Income (SSI) and is designed to help the aged, blind and disabled who have little or no income meet their basic needs such as food, clothing, and shelter. Although SSI is administered by the Social Security Administration, its funds come from the general fund not from moneys received from your Social Security taxes. You can apply for either online or by calling Social Security.

It is important to apply as soon as possible for all benefits. Social Security disability, for example, has a 6 month waiting period. In other words you must be disabled for 6 months to receive benefits. If you wait until you have been disabled that long, your benefits

Social Security's telephone number is 1-800-772-1213. Their web site for information on disabilities is www.ssa.gov/disability.

will not come to you until your application has been processed so you could be without funds for a long time.

Please note that both of these are federal programs.
Many states have their own disability programs. Although
they can piggyback onto the federal program, it is possible
to be certified disabled by the federal government and declined by the state and vice versa. It is also possible if you
have disability insurance, either privately or through your
employer, that your private insurer will grant disability and
the government won't, or the other way around. So apply
everywhere possible! Do not get discouraged if you are declined. Appeal if you believe your case has merit.

Social Security Death Benefit

Social Security pays survivors benefits to certain members of the family. Some widows and widowers, dependent
parents age 62 or over and some disabled children can receive survivors benefits. If a parent dies and meets certain
criteria, his/her children under the age of 18 may be eligible
to receive income from Social Security.

A spouse who is living with their partner at the time of
death is also entitled to a one time payment of $255. The
spouse may also be eligible for the last check or to receive
their spouse's regular Social Security depending on circumstances. Again, it is best to check directly with Social Security.

Medicaid/Medicare

Many people get these confused. Medicaid is a needs-
based program administered by individual states. Medicare
is a federal insurance program for people age 65 and over
if they or their spouse have worked the requisite amount of
time, some disabled people under the age of 65, and all
people with end-stage renal failure. People under 65 whom
the federal government has declared disabled for a period
of 2 years are eligible for Medicare.

Sometimes Medicaid will pay the Medicare premium for the disabled person. (This is a way to shuffle the primary cost for health care costs to the federal government.) Whereas Medicaid usually pays for all medical bills Medicare has a co-pay. Both will sometimes pay for durable medical equipment (DME) (see Chapter 4, "Knowledge is power" for more information about durable medical equipment). Some people with low incomes may be eligible for Medicaid only if they spend a certain amount monthly on medical bills. This amount varies with income and is known as a spend down. This means that before Medicaid will be effective, the person must have already spent a certain amount of his/her own money to pay for medical services. (Please note in recent years, some states have changed the name of Medicaid to make the name less confusing. For example, in New Hampshire some families can receive Medicaid for their children – the program is called Healthy Kids. Some low income-families can buy into the plan based on their income.)

If a child has a life threatening illness or disabling condition, he or she may be eligible for benefits from Medicaid. You should file an application as soon as the diagnosis is made. Again states differ in what they provide. It does not hurt to call for information or to apply as soon as possible.

Prescription Drug Coverage

If you do not have a public or private prescription drug coverage, are a legal resident of the United States or Puerto Rico, are not eligible for Medicare and meet certain household income levels, you may be able to use the Partnership for Prescription Assistance (www.pparx.org or call 1-888-4PPA-NOW (1-888-4772-669). This program is a collaborative effort of the pharmaceutical companies, doctors, and many organizations. It provides a single point of access to public and private programs for people who lack prescription drug coverage and who meet eligibility requirements. www.needymeds.com is another resource to find help with paying for medication.

Other Services Provided by Foundations and Non-profits

In many states there are other organizations which can assist caregivers or care receivers and provide an amazing menu of services. If you have a case manager or a social worker, she can often help you find that information. For example, a foundation in my state paid for a wheelchair ramp for someone who needed one but could not afford the cost. Usually, a number of telephone calls must be made to find out which foundation would do that. This is an opportunity to allow a good friend who has excellent telephone skills to be helpful (see Chapter 5, "Let me know if there is anything I can do for you" for other suggestions).

If the person is over the age of sixty-five, local Councils on Aging, Senior Centers or Area Agencies on Aging often have information about where services can be obtained. The National Council on Aging has a website to assist seniors in finding benefits; it is www.benefitscheckup. org. People with a particular disability may get help or information from the local or state chapter of an organization dedicated to that disability (See Chapter 4, "Knowledge is Power").

If the care recipient has a rare disease, there may be a national foundation dedicated to it. www.rarediseases.org lists rare diseases and the associations affiliated with them. The national organization for a particular disorder can often connect people to the best resources for that illness and may have a chat line as well. The National Institutes of Health also has a section on rare diseases, http://rarediseases.info. nih.gov/. A friend of mine with a rare disease participated in a study through the National Institute for Health but had to travel to Washington, DC for monitoring. www.nih.gov, their website, can provide you with information on all clinical trials. They also have a list of diseases which can provide information about the disease and its treatment. Sometimes people who live near large teaching hospitals can find a group of doctors dedicated to studying the problem. In these cases, usually the patient participates in research and receives medications and examinations free.

Foundations are non-profits and are usually quite helpful. If you have questions whether a particular foundation is legitimate or a scam, check with the Better Business Bureau, www.bbb.org. If you have a rare disease, your doctor's office may be able to provide you with legitimate resources.

Regardless of whether you are caring for someone who is facing a life-threatening illness, has a chronic condition or is disabled, there is probably an organization dedicated to it. That organization is your best source of information. However, there are many local and national foundations that provide support. Some offer financial support whereas others offer services. Many are restricted to a particular disease or region/state of the country. For example, the Weber Foundation in Melrose, Massachusetts provides financial assistance to individuals and their families who face life-threatening illnesses but their grants are limited to the northeastern states. The Make-a-Wish Foundation, on the other hand, is a national organization which grants wishes to children who have been diagnosed with a life-threatening illness. Again this is a great time to avail yourself of your friends who are good at tracking down information.

Trusts

If a spouse has become disabled, some couples have found it helpful to have any joint assets put in trust and/or to remove the disabled person's name from property ownership.

This is clearly a situation that requires legal advice and knowledge of your state's laws.

Fund Raising

When a sudden change in circumstance occurs, the financial repercussions make it challenging for us to provide for our families, pay mortgages, etc. and care for our loved one. Friends and communities often pitch in by having fund raisers or asking for donations. If you want funds paid into a non-profit and bills paid out of the non-profit, then you will need to go through the legal paperwork and procedures necessary to create a not-for-profit organization. An attorney may be necessary depending on state laws, your competency and time, and availability of friends who might help to complete and file the paperwork in a timely manner.

WORK

Check on flexible hours. More employers are becoming aware of the problems that beset caregivers and are willing to make accommodations. Your employer may prefer to have you work a schedule that allows you to be there most of the time or different hours rather than have to hire and train a new employee. Can you job share temporarily or on days when you need to? Can you telecommute, i.e. work from home on your computer or laptop?

Some employers hire per diem workers who are willing to come in and work when the normal staff is either out sick or on vacation. Perhaps someone who has recently retired from the job would be willing to pitch in on an occasional or even scheduled basis if it is okay with the employer.

In some workplaces, people may donate vacation time for people on family leave. (This was one of the best gifts I ever received when I was out for surgery!)

Most larger employers have an Employee Assistance Program (EAP) which is free and confidential to employees.

If you are unsure if your employer has one, you can check with human resources. EAPs offer a variety of services ranging from counseling to resource information to financial information. If you are a long distance caregiver, some can assist you in locating the connections needed to help place an elder or find other services.

Does your employer offer day care for adults or participate in a plan that you can join? Is there a day care near your home or work so that you can drop off the care recipient on your way to work and pick her up on the way home?

Be creative and ask. If your employer refuses, you are not any worse off than you were before. Maybe if you both put your heads together you can come up with a plan that will work for you and your employer. Remember it is to your employer's advantage to keep an employee rather than to hire and train a new one.

EDUCATION

If the loved one you are caring for is a child, the school district must make accommodations and modifications to assist your child. If your child is pre-school age or an infant, it is best to check with your pediatrician to verify your suspicions. If your doctor has already told you that your child has a disability, then you may contact your local school district to have a free evaluation to ascertain if your child is eligible for early intervention services. The National Dissemination Center for Children with Disabilities (www.nichcy.org or 1-800-695-0285) can provide you with additional information and a review of your rights.

FUNERALS/CREMATION/DONATING ORGANS & BODIES

If the prognosis is poor, then it can be helpful to discuss what the care recipient wishes to happen. As I mentioned in Chapter 1, Bob had made arrangements to donate his body to a medical school when he died so when he started hospice care I called them to verify the procedure. The coordinator asked me if I had alternate plans because they can't guarantee acceptance of the body. When I mentioned that Bob had made alternative arrangements through the NH Cremation Society, she suggested that I confirm it was an option and ascertain what they would provide.

I called them but they were a distance from where we were living and I would have to go there to get Bob's ashes. They would not provide any services such as giving the obituary to the papers or death certificates. Then, I called some local funeral homes closer to home. I was astounded at the variation in price; the most expensive was $4,000 more expensive than the closest and that did not include the urn for Bob's ashes. Since Bob was being cremated and there were not going to be calling hours or any service at the funeral home, I didn't understand the disparity.

When Bob died, the medical school was unable to accept his body. The coordinator did offer to see if hospitals in the adjoining states would accept the body but in one case I would have had to pay for the entire transportation of the body to the hospital and in the other, I would have to pay for transportation of the body to the state line. Since that would have been expensive, I chose to have Bob cremated. I felt sad that the school could not accept his body because Bob had gone there for all of his treatments and that would have been a way of giving back to them.

Some people indicate on their licenses that they wish to donate various organs. Again communication with family members and doctors is key. In order to harvest the organs, doctors must handle the death and body differently than they normally would.

It is difficult to have to deal with funeral and cremation arrangements when the caregiver is already stressed by the care recipient's pending or actual death. Therefore, I recommend exploring what options are available before it becomes necessary and then setting up the plan if the prognosis is poor and/or making arrangements so that the family does not have to worry about it Although you can prepay, you can also wait. If you opt to wait, you should let your family know what you wish done and with whom.

Bob had written his obituary prior to his becoming very ill. This was very helpful because it would have been extremely difficult for me or his children at the time of his death. Therefore, when possible, I recommend that the obituary also be written before the death. Simultaneously, you can decide which papers should print them.

Usually there is a fee to print obituaries based on the length and the fees of that paper. Most papers will print a death notice which simply tells the name and when and where someone died for free.

Discussing these issues can be challenging. Death is an emotionally charged subject and not everyone can face it calmly and reasonably. Talking about them can force us to face our own mortality. Family members may differ about what arrangements should be made. It may be easiest to do so before it is necessary. Step-families can encounter other opposition. In one family I know of, the spouse had asked his wife to handle his death a certain way but when he died his children refused to permit his request to be honored because he had not made it clear to them. Indeed this can occur in intact families. Making your wishes known and putting them in writing is a good way to proceed. After your wishes are put in writing and signed and dated by you, it is important that the family knows what they are and where to find the paper on which your wishes are written. It will prevent confusion and possibly conflict later.

LIFE INSURANCE

If the care recipient has life insurance, you will need to send a copy of the death certificate to the company. The company usually has another form to complete as well. I was shocked when I called them to see how much longer before I received my check. The person who answered told me that my account booklet and checks were on the way. Evidently, there was an option I missed when I completed the form or this insurance company handles it this way routinely. Basically what happened is the money I was entitled to had been put into an account in my name and held by the insurance company. They then sent me checks which I use to get any funds I might want. In my case the money was to earn 2.9% which at the time was better than I was getting at my bank for a savings account. I did have a choice at that time to have them then write a check or wait until I received my checks and write it for all or part of the amount. Our daughters did not encounter this problem with the insurance policy for which they were the beneficiaries.

VETERANS BENEFITS

No book would be complete without mentioning veterans, especially those who become care recipients and whose loved ones become caregivers. Veterans who have become disabled through serving in the armed services are eligible for medical services. Some who are not disabled may also be eligible for medical services. Since dates and lengths of service are important it is best to check directly with the Veterans Administration.

The Veterans Administration offers other benefits as well such as education, home loans, compensation and pension, vocational rehabilitation, life insurance and survivors benefits. This wide array of assistance can help the caregiver but it is important to become informed and advocate for those benefits for which you qualify. If the veteran has been discharged, you will need his discharge papers when filing for benefits.

http://www.arlingtoncem-etery.org/funeral_information/ guide.interment.html provides the eligibility requirements for burial at Arlington National Cemetery. For burial and memorial benefits provided by the Veterans Administration, see http://www.cem.va.gov/.

www.va.gov provides information about all of the benefits provided by the Veterans Administration or call the Veterans Benefits Service Center at 1-877-222-VETS (8387).

There are many financial supports out there but it is often a time-consuming and frustrating process discovering and taking advantage of them. States differ widely in what they provide and even locations within states can vary. Rural caregivers tend to have more challenges. People are becoming more aware of caregiving issues and Arizona, for example, has passed legislation to pass a Lifespan Respite Program. As awareness is raised about these difficult issues and its financial impact on those involved, other resources may become available.

CHAPTER 7

BEYOND ACCEPTANCE

Acceptance was a fragile state. When I came to terms with one facet of Bob's illness, another aspect reared its ugly head and there was a new challenge. At the same time, I was balancing a job, being a caregiver and trying to stay grounded in my spiritual beliefs.

Two of my beliefs are the power of prayer and the power of positive thinking. Research shows that prayer is helpful even if the person being prayed for has no knowledge of that prayer. When Bob was diagnosed with the tumor, I called my friends and each of them focused healing thoughts for Bob, sending positive energy and Light to him. We had Christians of various denominations, Jews, Muslims, Sufis, Hindus, Buddhists, and Bahais all centering their attentions on Bob and his health. This clearly worked. He did well beyond what most people expected. That is not to say it wasn't a struggle.

One of the worst weeks was when Bob developed pneumonia and pleurisy. We were staying in a room at our friend's condo. Martha took us in when we sold our home and had nowhere to live. I took Bob to the emergency room. They sent him home with medications. He was not sleeping well, was in considerable pain and was running a fever. I couldn't believe they sent him home and was afraid that Bob might have survived surgery and radiation, only to die of pneumonia. His pain and difficulty breathing impacted our rest. When he doesn't sleep well, I don't either. The following night I had to take Martha to the emergency room for her gall bladder. When I left Bob to take her to the hospital, I gave him instructions about what to do if his fever or pain increased hoping he understood and would comply. I finally arrived home at four in the morning because it took so long for the doctors to decide Martha needed to be admitted. I got up at my usual time of 6:30 a.m. and was at work by 8:00 a.m. making sure Bob had his medications and breakfast before I left. I functioned on autopilot. Fortunately, I knew what I had to do at work and eventually the antibiotics kicked in and Bob got better.

Those times did not leave any opportunity for reflection. It was like being on a ship during a storm at sea. The ship lists to port and starboard, while the bow rises up with the waves and then comes crashing down into the abyss created by those same waves. I never knew which way I would be thrown. When I thought I could take a step forward, I was pitched in another direction entirely. Maintaining balance is a challenge. Likewise, caregiving has ups and downs with no middles. I was always reacting to Bob's condition and symptoms, feeling that I wasn't living according to my spiritual beliefs. I wanted to be at peace within myself regardless of the tempest surrounding me.

My journey was about learning to surrender, to turn events and outcomes over to God without absolving me of responsibilities. Similar to the twelve step programs which state that there is a higher power and that there are

Serenity Prayer
   "God grant me the Serenity to accept the things I cannot change, Courage to change the things I can, And Wisdom to know the difference."
Reinhold Neibuhr

events over which I am powerless, I could pray, I could hope, I could believe, and I could wish. Even though I knew I didn't have the final say.

By turning over responsibility for Bob to Bob and to God, a Higher Power, or the Universe, I was only in charge of doing the best I could for both of us. That is all I could do anyway and, I might as well accept it.

When I had difficulty with these concepts I focused on the Serenity Prayer, trying to be the wise person who knew the difference between those things that I could control and those that I could not. It was not difficult to understand intellectually. The challenge was to live it in my heart. The highs came when he was well or at least better and the lows were when he was so sick. He would come through the surgery, the radiation, the pneumonia, etc. and I would feel better.

When Bob's condition stabilized, we planned for our future together. We moved to a new home where we could live on one floor. Although Bob was quite well then, I wasn't sure what the future held so I wanted to be prepared. We built our home so that it was wheelchair accessible in the event he had a reoccurrence. The day we moved, I was in the hospital for surgery and Bob was the well one.

His cancer did not return but the side effects from the brain tumor, the radiation and the surgery were on-going. Non-convulsive seizures, memory problems and confusion contributed to an unsteady existence. He worked hard around the house and on our property but his decisions were not always sound. It was a difficult balance between allowing him to live his life and being so strongly impacted by my own feelings.

Once when he wanted to build a miniature stonewall. My friend, Jane, and I watched as Bob worked on moving rock. He had very poor balance. We felt he was trying to do something that was beyond his capabilities and for which he did not have the correct equipment. Bob would try and move a stone with a system that he had jury-rigged and then lose his balance. Finally, when I could take no more, I became extremely concerned and angry. I told him to stop. I am sure he was embarrassed but he stopped. While I was at work the next day, he started the project again. When I returned home, he was extremely quiet and finally admitted he had hurt himself. Bob had fallen backwards onto the rock pile while trying to move a rock into place. He talked about getting up after he had rested and driving himself to the hospital to see if he had broken anything. I was irate. If he needed to go to the hospital, then we would go now. I wasn't going to let Bob get up in the night to drive himself to the hospital! I couldn't believe he would do that. I told him if he wanted to go I would take him. So I did.

I couldn't stop work to keep an eye on him and I couldn't control his behavior. He wasn't ill enough to be in an assisted living or nursing home, nor did I want this. I began to fear that one day I would come home from work and find him dead or badly injured. I wasn't sure which would be worse. For a while, this fear colored our lives. *When fear runs your life, you become paralyzed.* My decisions needed to be based on love not fear. I had to develop a plan to carry us into the future.

What helped me cope was deciding that he would be happier doing what he could and that he would rather die being active than sitting around feeling and being useless. His life, his choice. Of course, I realized that he could badly injure himself but that was the chance I was going to have to take. Initially, I could only intellectualize this but eventually through talking with friends, meditating, praying, writing about it, I accepted it emotionally as well. This was a difficult passage.

When I was sure I had come to terms with the idea, a couple of friends questioned whether or not we would like to renew our wedding vows. Bob and I decided we would like to and we had a recommitment ceremony, at which our friends officiated. It offered us a way to think about our future in spite of challenges. While I was talking with our friends a couple of months later, they pointed out it was still not okay with me for Bob to die. They felt I was holding on to him as though he were my life. And in some ways he was. I did not want him to die. I did not want to figure out how to live life without him. I did not want to mourn his passing. In fact, I did not even want to think about it! Yet I would get these constant reminders. It was as though the grim reaper was saying, "Okay, I spared him once but he's still mine and I can take him at anytime." Death was toying with me, letting me feel comfortable for a while and then scared for another while. I lost all serenity during these times.

My friends urged me not to hold onto him. One friend, Anna, said that she had found it necessary to do the same with her husband, Jim. Although Jim was not ill, he traveled a great deal. Every time he boarded a plane Anna worried and wondered. Finally, she felt that she could no longer deal with that stress and that she had to come to terms with whatever life held in store for both her and her husband. She expects and wants to have many more years with him and will mourn him when he dies but letting go took away her anxiety associated with every trip.

After this conversation, I began to realize that although I never wanted to deal with his passing I needed to come to terms with it – whether he died or not! Or, perhaps, regardless of when he died. Indeed, I could die first. I could not be dependent on his journey.

When we said our original wedding vows, we talked about two wholes coming together. During our time together we had fused so much into one another, or at least, I had melted into him. I needed to remember how to separate; I needed to relearn being whole. I would still grieve him terribly when he died but I would have accepted his death and his passing as his journey. I wanted another twenty plus years with him. But now I was willing to let him go if required. Without holding on.

When I first thought of this, the pain was unbearable. I wept for days and days, not being able to imagine life without him – not *wanting* to imagine life without him. The pain was emotional, physical, spiritual and mental. It was excruciating almost beyond what I could bear. I would be driving along the road and start to weep. I stormed, ranted and raved. Yelling out from pain, that I didn't want to do it, I didn't want to let him go. Yet always privately, with the exception of the first day when I had been with my friends, I couldn't bear to talk about it. It was a pain beyond sharing. Sharing would make it worse – more real – more devastating.

It was something I had to come to grips with myself.

Alone.

All alone.

Being alone and feeling that aloneness is one of the most demoralizing emotions one can try to contain in one's being. I am no exception. I knew that was part of my spiritual path and that if I went through the fire of pain, I would be stronger. Ultimately I would be able to let him go.

For days, I raged within myself. Wanting to say, not my will but Thine. Yet not ready to make that step.

Finally, on a bright, sunny day, I decided to go sit under the great-grandmother oak on our property. She has great strength and I've always seen her as the guardian of our property. I hoped she would give me strength for what I had to do.

I sat down on the ground, in lotus position for a specific meditation. I surrounded myself with a bubble of Love, Light, and Protection. I prayed to God for protection for my journey. I asked that my process be for everyone's highest and best good. I went into a meditative state. Then

I asked to go to in-between-time. When I arrived in my mind at in-between-time, I placed myself with Bob in the center of a square. At the corners of the square were my friends. I called on my family and friends, living and dead, as well as Bob's family who had already died to be there. Then, I walked with Bob to the threshold, the other side, where he would go when he dies. He was met by his parents with great joy. I was supported by friends. It seemed okay with me. But still I couldn't tolerate it for too long so I retrieved Bob and chose to end my meditative state. I was surprised at how good I felt, how right it was.

Until ...I felt the tears dropping on my legs. I realized my face was covered with tears which flowed in a torrent down my cheeks. I sat there for quite awhile until I began to get cold. So much for letting him go. I knew that I would need to do this meditation several times to complete the process.

Nevertheless a subtle shift occurred and our relationship seemed to soften towards each other. It's a bit like a tug of war where each is pulling in his own direction and when one stops, the war ends. I did not share this with Bob but I was sure he knew as he had so many times before.

I continued to practice the meditation and practice did make it easier. But mourning has its own process and takes its own time.

One day Bob shared that he had a nightmare in which he thought he was dying and that he had some things he needed to do first. Bob had already written his obituary, arranged for his body to be donated to a medical school or alternately, to be cremated. He wanted to make a list of people he wanted to invite to his memorial service. I wanted to know what he wanted in his memorial service – music, quotes, etc. He also had a project he was working on in the back yard that he wanted to see completed but a fallen tree which required removal by others impeded progress on it.

I believed since he had dreamt about dying his time might be near. I wanted his passage to be without stress since dying is difficult enough and the survival instinct is so strong. I started to work on these issues. God paved the way for many of my closest friends to move nearby shortly before Bob's dream. Simultaneously, I shared my thoughts, feelings and especially fears with them.

It is not comfortable to talk about a loved one's possible or impending death and often denial is the more common reaction. It reminds me of the dating dance – when one can talk about it, the other cannot; when the other is ready, the first is not. There may be moments when both can share the pain, the wonder, and the work. There is no right way.

A visit to the neurologist revealed that indeed it was a miracle for Bob to be alive after six years. I reveled in Bob's presence in my life. I focused on what he could do, his beautiful personality, and the fun times we continued to have. As I practiced acceptance of how he was, I also hoped for our future and prepared for when he died. These contradictory emotions and planning are all part of the caregiver's journey.

Bob had a couple of serious illnesses where he nearly died. In the first, he had an infection during which his temperature rose to 103.8 degrees. He was quite ill for nearly a week. The second illness was never really diagnosed. The doctors believed that he was having a delayed reaction to the whole brain radiation. Bob could not speak although he clearly understood what people said to him. Sometimes when he tried to talk only gibberish came out. Initially, doctors thought he might be having non-convulsive seizures because he seemed to improve during the day. He had difficulty walking and maintaining his balance. When the doctors felt they could do no more and it was a situation with which he would have to live, he was sent for rehabilitation at a skilled nursing facility, part of a nursing home, and he eventually improved.

When I saw Bob as sick and as frustrated as he was, I finally realized that it was finally okay with me for Bob to die. That did not mean that I would not mourn him, I still would. However, it was okay with me if he died. Interestingly when I reached that point I realized that my focus changed. I no longer thought about me. When I was going through denial, anger, depression, all of those emotions were about my feelings and me. After acceptance, my spotlight was on Bob. I noticed that I was no longer angry with him or his illness and its side effects. My care of him was kinder and more thoughtful. It enabled us to talk even more openly about what was happening to him. Bob said to a couple we knew well, "I don't think I'll be here next Christmas." Later on another day, he said, "I'm going soon." What was clear to me was that I didn't want him to suffer regardless of his time left.

Now our struggle evolved to maintaining his safety. I could no longer accept his need to do when in fact he couldn't. He, however, still wanted to and although I wanted him to do what he wanted, I had to deal with more injuries than I was able to comfortably. For example, one time I came home to find Bob in the shower with blood pouring out of his head. He was not aware of how badly injured he was. I knew scalp wounds bleed a lot but it was annoying to say the least. Only the next day when I showed him the stitches in the mirror did he say, "Oh, I guess it was good we went to the hospital." His dementia had reached the stage where he didn't always realize the extent of his injuries, particularly if he couldn't see them or feel them.

After Bob died, I realized that I had already processed much of my grief and was relieved. He was clearly frustrated by his inability to do and to talk. For someone whose livelihood had depended on his ability to speak before others, his deterioration was quite marked. People who saw him never gave me feedback about his condition which always surprised me. I'm not sure what I expected them to say or even what they could say. After he died, people remembered the good times which is as it should be.

Now I am concentrating on building a new life without him. I focus on Bob's death as a gift although there are still times when the waves of grief come crashing down on my equilibrium. Although this book is my contribution to other caregivers, it is also a way for me to find meaning in his illness and the mental anguish he experienced as a result of his tumor and treatment. Bob was a political junkie and helped to raise awareness about health care issues so ultimately this is his gift to all of you.

Take care.

GLOSSARY

Advance Care Planning – planning that families need to do with regard to healthcare, legal and financial issues (see Chapter VI, Finances and Legal Matters)

Brand name – see under drugs.

Caregiver – a person who is caring for a loved one who has been diagnosed with a life-threatening or chronic and debilitating illness or who has a disability

Care Recipient or Care Receiver - the loved one who is receiving care

CPR (Cardiopulmonary Resuscitation) – When there is no pulse and no breathing detected, this is the name given to reviving someone by using chest compressions and mouth to mouth breathing

Drugs – drugs are listed under two names, a brand name and a generic name. This can make if confusing. For example, Advil, Motrin, Nuprin and Medipren are all different brand names for the same drug, ibuprofen. If a drug company still holds the patent on a drug, there will only be the brand name of that company and the generic name. If the patent has expired, then all drug companies may manufacture the drug and promote it and the drug will have as many different names as drug companies manufacture it but the generic name will be the same for all of them.

Durable Medical Equipment – medical equipment that is not consumed or destroyed by use (see Chapter IV Knowledge is Power)

Durable Power of Attorney for Health Care - a document in which you name the person you trust to make healthcare decisions for you if you are unable to.

Do Not Resuscitate (DNR) – an order given by your doctor which states that you do not want any attempt to restart either your breathing or your heart if either has stopped.

Generic Name – for explanation look under drugs

Health Care Agent - the person named in the durable power of attorney for health care to act for you

Health Care Proxy - same as durable power of attorney for health care

Hospice - a program that provides services to people who are nearing the end of their life and support to their families. The patient can be at home, or at a facility. Hospitals and nursing homes often have beds designated for that purpose.

Living Will – a document which conveys your wishes about life-sustaining treatments if you are unable to speak for yourself or are permanently unconscious.

Metastasis – the spread of a disease from one part of the body to another, usually referred to in cancer. A cancer that has spread is usually far more challenging to treat.

Palliative care – is intended to relieve pain. Although often associated with hospice, palliative care is its own specialty. Its goal is relieve pain and provide the best possible quality of life for anyone who is in pain, regardless of diagnosis or prognosis.

Prognosis – a prediction about the probable course of the disease.

APPENDIX

Advance Directives

www.uslivingwillregistry.com is a web site dedicated to living wills. It provides forms, connections to the American Bar Association and the ability to register your advance directive on their site through one of their community partners.

www.putitinwriting.org explains about advance directives. It provides a link to individual state information, a glossary of terms, and an individual card that you can print out and carry in your wallet so that health care providers will know that you have an advance directive.

www.compassionandchoices.org was formed when two organizations, Compassion in Dying and End-of-Life Choices, merged. It is the largest organization in the United States advocating for patients' rights at the end of life. Under the services heading, click on Living Wills to get information about advance directives. Or you may call at 1-800-247-7421. They will also assist you if you are having difficulty having your advance directive honored. Its services are free and funded by donations and memberships.

Non-computer options. If you do not have a computer or do not have access to a computer, you can check with your primary care physician's office or the nearest hospital.

Caregiver Organizations

Share the Care. www.sharethecare.org/ is a web site and a book about how to organize a group of people to care for someone who is seriously ill. sharethecaregiving, Inc., 551 Fifth Avenue - 28th Floor, New York, NY 10176 is the mailing address. 646 467-8097 is the only telephone number given.

Family Caregiver Alliance (FCA). www.caregiver.org is "dedicated to family caregivers and the professionals who help them and to increase public awareness of issues facing family caregivers." They have an extensive list of fact sheets, reading lists, etc. – they range from free to costly. They have a newsletter to which you can subscribe. Their address is Family Caregiver Alliance, 180 Montgomery St., Ste 1100, San Francisco, CA 94104 and their toll free is 1-800-445-8106.

National Family Caregivers Association (NFCA). www. nfcacares.org "supports, empowers and speaks up for caregivers," They hope to minimize the disparity between caregivers and non-caregivers. They pushed for The National Family Caregiver Support Program, federal legislation to address family caregivers, which will work through Area Agencies on Aging to provide counseling, respite, information and referral services. They offer a free, quarterly publication to family caregivers and can be reached through their website (see above), at 10400 Connecticut Avenue, Suite 500,Kensington, MD 20895-3944 or toll free at1-800-896-3650. Others including former caregivers interested in caregiving can also receive the newsletter but there is a fee.

National Caregiving Foundation. www.caregiving-foundation.org focuses primarily on caring for Alzheimer's patients and will send a Caregiver Support Kit to caregiver's free of charge. Their toll free number is 1-800-930-1357.

AARP's Caregiving Resource. www.aarp.org/caregivinghelp1 is a resource that provides lots of information for caregivers of older people. It includes strategies for self-care, resources, and connections with other caregivers.

Hospice Organizations

Hospice Foundation of America (HFA) www.hospicefoundation.org is intended to help people who "must cope personally or professionally with terminal illness, death, and the process of grief and bereavement." They provide excellent information about hospice and how it can help the dying. They may be reached at (800) 854-3402. They sponsor an annual teleconference related to issues of grief.

www.hospicenet.org is a web site for patients and families facing a life-threatening illness. It has links for services, patients, caregivers, children and bereavement. Under services, there is a link to find a local hospice.   However, it does not have an 800 number so a computer is a must. Their mailing address is Hospice, Suite 51, 401 Bowling Avenue, Nashville, TN 375025-5124.

www.caringinfo.org is the web site of "Caring Connections, a program of the National Hospice and Pallaitive Care Organization (NHPCO), and is a national consumer engagement initiative to improve care at the end of life, supported by a grant from the Robert Wood Johnson Foundation." From their web site you can access the advance directives for each state. They have a toll free number, 800-658-8898, which provides information about end-of-life care and will send appropriate brochures.

If you do not have access to a computer, look in your telephone book under hospice or palliative care. If there is no listing, call a local visiting nurse organization or the nearest hospital.

Disease Related Web Sites

www.webmd.com can provide general information about common diseases and terminology.

www.rarediseases.org provides information about rare disorders.

Prescription Drug Programs

www.pparx.org is a web site that helps people who do not have prescription drug coverage to help coordinate programs that may provide necessary medications at little or no cost.

Respite Resources

Family Caregiver Alliance – www.caregiver.org provides a state-by-state listing of respite services for family caregivers.

National Easter Seal Society – www.easterseals.org offers children and adults with disabilities home services, camps and adult day programs. (1-800-221-6827)

Check with state agencies for local information or the volunteer organization that deals with the particular diagnosis the care recipient has such as the American Cancer Society or the Brain Injury Association.

Volunteer Organizations

Corporate Angel Network is based in White Plains, NY and "arranges free travel on corporate jets for cancer patients, bone marrow donors and bone marrow recipients as long as they: travel to or from an approved cancer treatment center, are able to walk up and down the steps to a private plane without assistance, and do not require oxygen, IV or any other form of life support during the flight." Children are permitted to travel with two adults. Their toll-free patient line is 866-328-1313. They suggest that a patient make back-up travel arrangements because they cannot guarantee the ability to find a flight that matches the patient's needs. www.corpangelnetwork.org can provide additional information.

GUIDED IMAGERY

Guided imagery is a technique similar to meditation that helps us to relax thus decreasing stress. You do not need to know how to meditate. It does use your imagination and senses. If you are one of those people who can see things, then use that ability. For example, if you are out somewhere, could you close your eyes and "see your kitchen?" If so, you can visualize things. Perhaps you're a feeler. You enjoy feeling the textures – soft, hard, wet, dry, fuzzy, etc. Musicians have acute hearing and can often hear music in their heads. Whichever sense of our five senses you can use during the process will help. Employ more than one if you can.

The best way to use the following is to read it through once and then record it so you can play it back without having to read it. The next option is to have someone read it to you. It should be read slowly, softly and quietly. I have left spaces between the lines intentionally so that the reader will pause between each line.

If possible, dim the lights in your room. Although often calming music is helpful, I don't recommend it because I have found that music we like and think is appropriate when we try to use it for this process, the rhythm is off or it is louder than we think. Additionally, music which may soothe some may be disconcerting or annoying to others.   Under no circumstances do this when you are driving or operating any kind of machinery.

If the first few times you do this, "nothing happens." That is okay. At least you have taken a few quiet moments for yourself and that in itself can be helpful. Just keep doing the process.

After you have completed the guided imagery, take a few moments to center yourself in the room and be sure to drink plenty of water throughout the day.

I have provided two different scripts for you. This will allow you to pick one and stick with it, or try both and see which is more effective for you, or to alternate them depending on how you are feeling. To do these, you should find a comfortable chair, preferably one with a straight back. Get comfortable in your chair, if possible do not cross your arms or legs during this process. If you are religious, you can say the Lord's Prayer prior to beginning. If not, repeat a mantra like om-m-m-m a number of times before you begin and ask that you be protected.

Guided Imagery #1

Close your eyes and imagine the brightest, whitest Light about a foot above your head.

Imagine that the white Light flows from the object directly into your head and fills your entire head cavity with that Light.

The Light continues to flow down your shoulders ...
down through the chest cavity...
filling the entire chest cavity

Continuing down through your abdomen.....

by now the entire upper part of your body is surrounded and filled with this bright, white Light.

This Light continues to flow down through your lower body...

through your hips......

your legs.

Out your feet and into the ground.

The Light at your shoulders flows down into your upper arms...

into your lower arms...

through your hands and out your hands back to the source.

(Sit and enjoy this flowing Light for about a minute.)

Now imagine that you see this table sitting in a beautiful green meadow.

You walk over to the table and you notice a gold box sitting on the table.

Next to the gold box is a pad of paper and a pencil

On the pad of paper you write down any concerns, worries, anxieties, struggles, things you think you may have done wrong in caring for your loved one....

(Pause)

When you are finished writing your list, tear off the list from the pad and place the list in the box and imagine that every item on that list is being put into the box.

(Pause)

You notice beyond the meadow a vast body of water and a small sail boat that is just large enough to hold your box. Place your box on the sail boat and push it out into the water.

A wave comes and takes the boat out. You watch as the boat gets smaller and smaller.

Finally, you cannot see the boat any longer ....

And you realize that you are no longer weighed down by anything that was on the list.

You feel as though a weight has been lifted off of your shoulders.

(Pause)

You continue to sit there for a while enjoying this feeling of peace and serenity.

(longer pause – about 1 minute)

You know that you can come back and enjoy this serenity anytime you want.

Now it is time to come back into the room.

Slowly open your eyes.

Guided Imagery #2

Close your eyes and get comfortable in your seat.

Imagine a bright gold ball about a foot below your feet.

The gold from that ball comes up into your feet filling them with its beautiful golden Light.

Imagine the gold Light continuing to flow up your body...

up your legs to your knees...

Continuing on up to your thighs and hips...

Into your abdomen.....

Filling your chest cavity with its bright Light...

Up your neck into your head...down your shoulders

Down your arms and out your hands

Then the Light continues up through your head to another gold ball about a foot above your head...

The gold light from the ball above your head forms a beautiful waterfall of gold Light that surrounds you and protects you as it envelops you in its Light...

Falling and returning to the gold ball below your feet.

So that now you are enclosed in a giant bubble of gold Light.

Relish that feeling for a while. (about a minute)

You feel very peaceful and serene

It feels so good to relax and enjoy it for a bit.

If there is any tension in your body, just imagine the gold Light filling that area and taking away your stress.

(Pause – about 1 minute)

Now you hear a quiet, gentle voice saying, "you are a good caregiver."

"You are doing the best you can."

Relax into the gentleness of the voice. (pause)

It feels so good to be in the gold Light...

To know that you are a wonderful, thoughtful caregiver...

(pause about ½ minute)

You are really enjoying this opportunity and relaxation.

You deserve it.

You work hard every day.

(Just enjoy this feeling for awhile...)

Know that you can return and recapture this feeling any time you want.

Know that you are loved.

(pause)

When you are ready, you may gradually come back into the room and open your eyes.

Some people do not notice any difference the first few times they do these processes. Like anything else it does require practice. One of the keys is to say it quietly and slowly and to do it when you know you will not be disturbed and to listen to it. It is not effective if you are trying to read it and imagine it. You may also download a copy of each from my website, www.joanperry.net.

www.ingramcontent.com/pod-product-compliance
Lightning Source LLC
Chambersburg PA
CBHW021955170526
45157CB00003B/996